796·07

STUDENT UNIT GUIDE

NEW EDITION

AQA AS Physical Education Unit 1

Opportunities for, and the Effects of, Leading a Healthy and Active Lifestyle

Symond Burrows, Michaela Byrne

and Sue Young

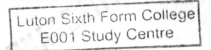
Philip Allan, an imprint of Hodder Education, an Hachette UK company, Market Place, Deddington, Oxfordshire OX15 0SE

Orders

Bookpoint Ltd, 130 Milton Park, Abingdon, Oxfordshire OX14 4SB

tel: 01235 827827

fax: 01235 400401

e-mail: education@bookpoint.co.uk

Lines are open 9.00 a.m.–5.00 p.m., Monday to Saturday, with a 24-hour message answering service. You can also order through the Philip Allan Updates website: www.philipallan.co.uk

© Symond Burrows, Michaela Byrne and Sue Young 2012

ISBN 978-1-4441-7138-9

First printed 2012
Impression number 5 4 3 2 1
Year 2017 2016 2015 2014 2013 2012

Cover photo: Fotolia

Typeset by Integra Software Services Pvt. Ltd., Pondicherry, India

Printed in Dubai

Hachette UK's policy is to use papers that are natural, renewable and recyclable products and made from wood grown in sustainable forests. The logging and manufacturing processes are expected to conform to the environmental regulations of the country of origin.

Contents

Content Guidance

Questions & Answers

Getting the most from this book

Questions & Answers

Exam-style questions

Examiner comments on the questions
Tips on what you need to do to gain full marks, indicated by the icon ⓔ.

Sample student answers
Practise the questions, then look at the student answers that follow each question.

Examiner commentary on sample student answers
Find out how many marks each answer would be awarded in the exam and then read the examiner comments (preceded by the icon ⓔ) following each student answer.

Structured questions   Section A

Section A **Structured questions**

Applied exercise physiology

Question 1

Health, exercise and fitness

(a) **Identify two components of fitness that are required by a sprint swimmer. Give an example of how one of these components is used in a race.** (3 marks)

ⓔ Make sure you identify two components of fitness as well as explaining how one of them is used in the race.

(b) **In a football game it is important for the performer to be fit and healthy. What do you understand by the terms fitness and health? Discuss whether you must be healthy in order to be fit.** (3 marks)

Total: 6 marks

ⓔ Make sure you give two definitions as well as looking at the link between health and fitness.

Student A
(a) Speed   and reaction time

ⓔ 2/3 marks awarded Having correctly identified two fitness components required by a sprint swimmer, the student forgets to say how one of these components is used during a race. Always read the question carefully and check your answer. Look at the number of marks available — this indicates the number of points you need to make.

Student B
(a) Speed   and power   . Power is needed to get off the blocks with as much force as possible   .

ⓔ 3/3 marks awarded The student correctly names two relevant fitness components required by a sprint swimmer and then says when one of these is important in a race. Always choose the fitness components that are most relevant to the sporting activity asked for.

Student A
(b) Fitness is the ability to cope with the demands of the environment   and being healthy means having a good social, mental and physical wellbeing   . Fitness is to do with the components such as speed and reaction time, whereas health is more medical.

Unit 1: Opportunities for, and the Effects of, Leading a Healthy and Active Lifestyle   81

About this book

This unit guide is written to help you prepare for the AQA PE Unit 1 test. **Section A** of the Unit 1 test examines the AS theoretical content of three aspects of PE, namely:
- applied exercise physiology
- skill acquisition
- opportunities for participation

The question in **Section B** relates to the practical aspects of applied skill and fitness and training, which are outlined in Unit 2 of the AS specification.

Each aspect of the specification required for the Unit 1 test is covered in the **Content Guidance** section, which summarises the key information that you need to understand and apply in the test. This section also includes examiner tips on what you will be expected to be able to do. Remember that this section is designed to *support* your revision, therefore it should be used in conjunction with your textbook, your own revision notes and other resources.

The **Questions & Answers** section of this guide provides examples of questions from various topic areas, together with student answers and examiner comments on how these could have been improved.

Content Guidance

Applied exercise physiology

Health, exercise and fitness

Definitions of fitness and health

Fitness can be difficult to define because it means different things to different people. One generic definition of fitness is: the ability to perform daily tasks without undue fatigue.

These daily tasks will be quite different for a non-athletic person compared with an elite performer. The fitness requirements of physical activities also vary. For example, the 100 metres sprint requires the body to work anaerobically with great strength, speed and power, whereas the marathon requires good muscular endurance and excellent aerobic capacity.

Health is often defined as a state of complete physical, mental and social wellbeing, and not merely the absence of disease or infirmity.

Examiner tip
Make sure you understand the relationship between health and fitness — you can be fit and healthy as well as fit and unhealthy.

Components of fitness

- Components of health-related fitness include cardiorespiratory endurance (also called stamina, VO_2(max) or aerobic capacity), muscular endurance, maximum strength, static strength, explosive strength, speed, power and flexibility.
- Components of skill-related fitness include agility, reaction time, coordination and balance.

Definitions of the components of fitness are given in Tables 1 and 2.

Table 1 Health-related components

Component	Definition
Cardiorespiratory endurance (stamina)	The ability to take in and use oxygen during prolonged exercise to delay the onset of fatigue
Muscular endurance	The ability of a muscle to perform repeated contractions and withstand fatigue
Maximum strength	The maximum force a muscle can exert in a single voluntary contraction
Static strength	Holding a position by muscles maintaining a state of contraction
Explosive strength	Rapid contraction of muscle fibres to achieve maximum force (related to power)
Speed	How fast a person can move a specified distance or how quickly a body part can be put into motion

Power	The amount of work performed per unit of time. It is the product of strength and speed
Static flexibility	Range of movement around a joint
Dynamic flexibility	Resistance of a joint to movement

Table 2 Skill-related components

Component	Definition
Agility	Ability to move and position the body quickly and effectively while under control
Reaction time	The time taken from detection of a stimulus to the initiation of a response
Coordination	The ability of the motor and nervous systems to interact so that motor tasks can be performed more accurately
Balance	The ability to keep the centre of mass over the base of support. It can be static, such as a handstand, or dynamic, where balance is retained in motion

Effect of lifestyle choices on health and fitness

Individuals make choices in life and these can have an effect on both health and fitness. For example, a poor diet can lead to obesity and health complications; smoking can affect the efficiency of oxygen transport; a lack of exercise can lead to heart and mobility problems; alcohol can affect concentration levels and make you less alert and, in excess, can damage the heart.

Knowledge check 1
What do you understand by the term 'power'?

Examiner tip
As well as defining each component of fitness, make sure you can apply each of these components to different sports.

Knowledge check 2
Explain how lifestyle choices can negatively affect performance in endurance sports.

After studying this topic, you should be able to:
- define health and fitness and understand the relationship between them and the problems associated in their definition
- understand the effects of lifestyle choices on health and fitness
- define the health-related components of fitness: stamina, muscular endurance, strength, speed, power and flexibility
- define the skill-related components of fitness: agility, reaction time, coordination and balance

Summary

Nutrition

The seven classes of food

Carbohydrates

Simple carbohydrates are found in fruit and are easily digested by the body. They are also present in many processed foods and anything with refined sugar added. **Complex carbohydrates** are found in nearly all plant-based foods, and usually take longer for the body to digest. They are most commonly found in bread, pasta, rice and vegetables.

Carbohydrate is an important source of energy during activity, and it is the main source of energy during high-intensity exercise. Carbohydrates are stored in the muscle and liver as glycogen and transported in the form of glucose. They store a lot of energy and should be consumed before, during and after exercise.

It is important to consider the glycaemic index (release rate) of different carbohydrates and the consequence this has on *when* they should be consumed in relation to training. Foods with a low glycaemic index cause a slow, sustained release of glucose to the blood, whereas foods with a high glycaemic index cause a rapid, sharp rise in blood glucose. Suitable foods to eat 3–4 hours before exercise include beans on toast, pasta or rice with a vegetable-based sauce, breakfast cereal with milk, or crumpets with jam or honey. Suitable snacks to eat 1–2 hours before exercise include fruit smoothies, cereal bars, fruit-flavoured yoghurt and fruit. An hour before exercise, liquid consumption appears to be more important — for example, sports drinks and cordials.

Fats

Fats are the secondary energy fuel for low-intensity aerobic work such as jogging and are made from glycerol and fatty acids. Fats contain a high proportion of carbon, which is why they give us so much energy, and they are also a good source of vitamins A, D, E, and K. Fats are stored in the muscle as triglycerides and transported as fatty acids.

Proteins

Proteins consist of chains of amino acids. They are important for tissue growth and repair and to make enzymes, hormones and haemoglobin. Proteins in the muscles may start to be broken down to provide energy when glycogen and fat stores are low, such as during strenuous activities or sustained periods of exercise.

Vitamins

Vitamins are needed for muscle and nerve functioning, tissue growth and the release of energy from foods. Vitamins cannot be stored in the body and excess amounts are excreted through urine.

Minerals

Minerals assist in bodily functions. For example, calcium is important for strong bones and teeth, and iron helps form haemoglobin, which is needed for the transport of oxygen and therefore to improve stamina levels. Minerals tend to be dissolved by the body as ions and are called electrolytes. These facilitate the transmission of nerve impulses and enable effective muscle contraction, both of which are important during exercise. However, it is important to get the right balance — too much sodium (contained in salt) can result in high blood pressure. As with vitamins, excessive consumption is unlikely to enhance performance.

Knowledge check 3

Give two classes of food suitable for a games player.

Fibre

Good sources of fibre are wholemeal bread and pasta, potatoes, nuts, seeds, fruit, vegetables and pulses. Fibre is important during exercise as it can slow down the time it takes the body to break down food, which results in a slower, more sustained, release of energy.

Water

Water constitutes approximately 60% of a person's body weight and is essential for good health. It carries nutrients to cells in the body and removes waste products. It also helps to control body temperature. When an athlete starts to exercise, production of water increases (water is a by-product of the aerobic system). We also lose a lot of water through sweat. The volume of water lost depends on the external temperature, the intensity and duration of the exercise and the volume of water consumed before, during and after exercise. Water is important to maintain optimal performance. Sports drinks such as Lucozade Sport and Gatorade can boost glucose levels before and after competition, while water rehydrates during competition.

A balanced diet

A balanced diet should contain 15% protein, 30% fat and 55% carbohydrate. For athletes in training, the percentage of carbohydrate should be increased. Sports nutritionists recommend:

- 10–15% protein
- 15–25% fat
- 60–75% carbohydrate

The energy balance of food

Energy is obtained from the food we eat (or from what the body stores). It is measured in calories. A calorie (cal) is the amount of heat energy required to raise the temperature of 1 g of water by 1°C. A kilocalorie (kcal) is the amount of heat required to raise the temperature of 1000 g of water by 1°C.

The basic energy requirement of an average person is generally given as 1.3 kcal per hour per kilogram of body weight. So someone who weighs 60 kg requires 1.3 × 24 (hours in a day) × 60 = 1872 kcal per day.

The energy requirement increases during exercise to 8.5 kcal per hour for each kilogram of body weight. So in a 1-hour training session the performer needs an extra 8.5 × 1 × 60 = 510 kcal. The total daily energy requirement of this performer is therefore 1872 + 510 = 2382 kcal.

What should you eat before a competition?

A pre-competition meal should be eaten 3–4 hours before competing because the food needs to be digested and absorbed in order to be useful. The meal needs to be high in carbohydrate, low in fat and moderate in fibre, to aid digestion (foods high in fat, protein and fibre tend to take longer to digest). High levels of carbohydrate will keep the blood glucose levels high throughout the competition/performance.

Examiner tip

Make sure you know the exercise-related function of each food type, e.g. fats are a good energy source for aerobic/low-intensity exercise and a good source of vitamins A, D, E and K.

Knowledge check 4

What do you understand by the term 'balanced diet'?

Diet of an endurance athlete versus a power athlete

The body's preferred fuel for endurance sport is muscle glycogen. If glycogen stores become depleted, the athlete becomes fatigued and is unable to maintain the intensity of training. To replenish and maintain glycogen stores, endurance athletes need a diet rich in carbohydrates — at least 6–10 grams of carbohydrate per kilogram of body weight per day. Water is also essential, to avoid dehydration.

Examiner tip

Questions will ask you to compare the diets of a power athlete and endurance athlete, but make sure you also know *why* power athletes eat more protein and endurance athletes eat more carbohydrates.

Some endurance athletes manipulate their diet to maximise aerobic energy production. One method is **glycogen loading**, which is covered at A2.

Endurance athletes require more carbohydrates and fats than power athletes because they exercise for longer periods of time and need more energy. Protein is very important for power athletes. Insufficient protein leads to muscle breakdown. Protein is necessary for tissue growth and repair.

Body fat composition

This is the physiological make-up of an individual in terms of the distribution of lean body mass and body fat. On average, men have less body fat (15%) than women (25%). Less body fat generally means a better performance. However, some sports have specific requirements for large amounts of fat, for example the defensive linesman in American football and sumo wrestlers.

Body mass index (BMI)

Body mass index (BMI) takes into account body composition. To calculate BMI, a person's weight in kilograms is divided by his/her height (in metres) squared. For example, a person who is 1.80 m tall weighing 75 kg has a BMI of $75/(1.8 \times 1.8) = 23.15$.

BMI classifications vary but the following is representative of most literature:
- **BMI < 19**   underweight
- **BMI 19–25**   normal
- **BMI 25–30**   overweight
- **BMI 30–40**   obese
- **BMI > 40**   morbidly obese

Obesity and limitations of definition

Obesity is an excess proportion of total body fat, usually due to energy intake being greater than energy output. Obesity carries an increased risk of heart disease, hypertension, high blood cholesterol, stroke and diabetes. It increases stress on joints and limits flexibility.

An individual is considered to be obese when his/her body weight is 20% or more above normal weight, or when a male accumulates 25% and a female 35% total body fat. The body mass index can also be used as a measure of obesity. An individual is considered obese when his/her BMI is over 30.

Knowledge check 5

Identify two diseases associated with obesity.

After studying this topic, you should be able to:
- list the seven classes of food and understand the exercise-related function of each food type
- describe a balanced diet and the energy balance of food, and be able to relate this to your own practical activity
- identify the difference in diet composition between endurance athletes and power athletes
- identify the percentage of body fat/body composition and body mass index (BMI) as measures of nutritional suitability
- give a definition of obesity and understand the limitations in trying to define it

Summary

Pulmonary function

The mechanics of breathing

Air moves from areas of high pressure to areas of low pressure. The greater the pressure difference, the faster air flows.

Changing the volume of the thoracic cavity alters the pressure of air in the lungs. **Inspiration** increases the volume of the thoracic cavity through contraction of the muscles surrounding the lungs. This reduces the pressure of air in the lungs. **Expiration** decreases the volume of the thoracic cavity. This increases the pressure of air in the lungs, forcing air out. At rest, expiration is a passive process. The muscles involved in respiration are given in Table 3.

Knowledge check 6

During a game of football, name the extra muscles used during inspiration.

Table 3 Respiratory muscles

Ventilation phase	Muscles used during breathing at rest	Muscles used during exercise
Inspiration	Diaphragm	Diaphragm
	External intercostals	• External intercostals • Sternocleidomastoid • Scalenes • Pectoralis major
Expiration	Diaphragm and external intercostals relax (passive process)	• Internal intercostals • Abdominals

Respiratory volumes

Definitions and values of respiratory volumes, and the way they change during exercise, are given in Table 4.

Table 4

Lung volume or capacity	Definition	Average values at rest (litres)	Change during exercise
Tidal volume	Volume of air breathed in *or* out per breath	0.5	Increase
Inspiratory reserve volume	Volume of air that can be forcibly inspired after a normal breath	3.1	Decrease
Expiratory reserve volume	Volume of air that can be forcibly expired after a normal breath	1.2	Slight decrease
Residual volume	Volume of air that remains in the lungs after maximum expiration	1.2	No change
Vital capacity	Volume of air forcibly expired after maximum inspiration in one breath	4.8	No change
Minute ventilation	Volume of air breathed in or out per minute	6	Large increase
Total lung capacity	Vital capacity + residual volume	6	No change

Examiner tip
Questions usually ask for definitions of tidal volume, inspiratory reserve volume and expiratory reserve volume, together with an explanation of what happens to these volumes during exercise.

Lung capacities can be measured from a spirometer trace (see Figure 1).

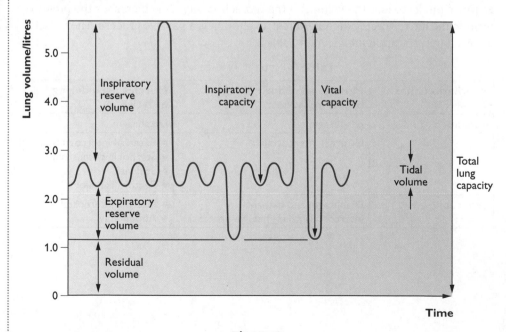

Figure 1

Gaseous exchange at the lungs

Gaseous exchange at the lungs is concerned with the replenishment of oxygen in the blood and the removal of carbon dioxide.

Diffusion is the movement of a gas from an area of high concentration to an area of low concentration down a concentration gradient until equilibrium is reached. In the lungs, diffusion of gases is aided by the structure of the alveoli. Alveoli are only one cell thick, so there is a short diffusion pathway; they have a vast surface area, which facilitates diffusion; and they are surrounded by a dense network of capillaries. The rate of diffusion is approximately 250 cm^3 of oxygen per minute at rest but this can rise to over 5 litres of oxygen per minute during exercise.

Oxygen makes up approximately 21% of air, so it exerts a partial pressure. Gases flow from areas of high pressure to areas of low pressure. As oxygen moves from the alveoli to the blood and then to the muscle, its partial pressure in each has to be successively lower.

The exchange of gases in the lungs takes place between alveolar air and blood flowing through the lung (pulmonary) capillaries. Oxygen enters the blood from the alveoli because the partial pressure of oxygen in the alveoli (105 mmHg) is higher than the partial pressure of oxygen in the incoming blood vessels (40 mmHg). This is because the working muscles remove oxygen, so its concentration in the blood is lower and therefore so is its partial pressure. The difference between any two pressures is referred to as the pressure gradient and the steeper this gradient, the faster diffusion will be. Oxygen diffuses from the alveoli into the blood until the pressure is equal in both.

The movement of carbon dioxide occurs similarly but from the blood to the alveoli, because the partial pressure of carbon dioxide in the blood is higher (46 mmHg) than that in the alveoli (40 mmHg).

Inspired air contains more oxygen than expired air; expired air contains more carbon dioxide than inspired air. The percentage concentrations of gases found in inspired and expired air are shown in Table 5.

> **partial pressure** the pressure exerted by an individual gas when it exists within a mixture of gases

Table 5

	Inspired air (%)	Expired air at rest (%)	Expired air during exercise (%)
Oxygen	21	16.4	15
Carbon dioxide	0.03	4	6

Gaseous exchange at the tissues

This takes place between arterial blood, flowing through the tissue capillaries, and the cells. Oxygen diffuses out of the arterial blood and into the muscle cells because the partial pressure of oxygen is higher (100 mmHg) in the blood than in the cells (40 mmHg).

Arterio-venous difference

This is the difference between the oxygen content of the arterial blood arriving at the muscles and the venous blood leaving the muscles. At rest, the arterio-venous difference is low because the muscles do not require much oxygen. However, during exercise the muscles need more oxygen, so the arterio-venous difference is high. This increase in A-VO$_2$ affects gaseous exchange at the alveoli. There is a higher concentration of carbon dioxide and a lower level of oxygen in the venous blood returning to the heart (and then being sent to the lungs). This increases the diffusion gradient of both gases.

Training also increases the arterio-venous difference, because trained performers can extract more oxygen from the blood.

Figure 2 highlights the differences in the partial pressure of oxygen and carbon dioxide in the alveoli, blood and muscle cells, and shows the A-VO$_2$ difference.

Figure 2

Transport of oxygen

Only about 3% of oxygen dissolves in plasma; approximately 97% combines with **haemoglobin** to form **oxyhaemoglobin**. When fully saturated, each haemoglobin molecule carries four oxygen molecules. At the tissues, oxygen dissociates from haemoglobin because of the lower pressure of oxygen in the tissues. In the muscle cells, oxygen is taken up by myoglobin. This has a high affinity for oxygen, which means that it can act as an oxygen store. During exercise, there is increased cellular respiration. As a result, the partial pressure of oxygen in the cell decreases to the point where myoglobin gives up its oxygen to the mitochondria.

The relationship of oxygen and haemoglobin can be represented by the oxyhaemoglobin dissociation curve (see Figure 3).

Examiner tip

Make sure you can define A-VO$_2$ difference and explain that it increases during exercise.

Knowledge check 7

Explain how oxygen is transported in the blood.

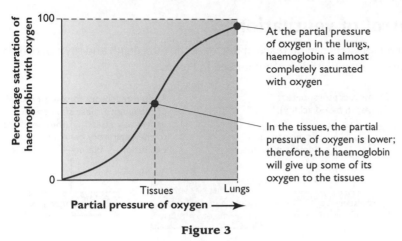

At the partial pressure of oxygen in the lungs, haemoglobin is almost completely saturated with oxygen

In the tissues, the partial pressure of oxygen is lower; therefore, the haemoglobin will give up some of its oxygen to the tissues

Figure 3

During exercise, this S-shaped curve shifts to the right because there is an increased demand for oxygen. Exercise creates conditions that cause haemoglobin to release some of its oxygen more readily. These conditions are:

- an increase in temperature in the blood and muscle
- a decrease in the partial pressure of oxygen in the muscle, which increases the oxygen diffusion gradient
- an increase in carbon dioxide in the blood, which increases the carbon dioxide diffusion gradient
- an increase in blood acidity (lower pH), which causes oxygen to dissociate from haemoglobin more quickly (Bohr effect, see Figure 4)

Examiner tip
Questions usually ask you to say what happens to the oxyhaemoglobin dissociation curve (it shifts to the right) and explain why this occurs.

Low carbon dioxide (at rest)

High carbon dioxide (during exercise)

In the tissues there is a low partial pressure of oxygen and high partial pressure of carbon dioxide, so haemoglobin unloads at this point — even more oxygen is available to the tissues

Figure 4

A question on control of breathing may refer to how an increase in carbon dioxide can affect breathing.

Control of ventilation

The nervous system can increase or decrease the rate, depth and rhythm of breathing. The control of ventilation is summarised in Figure 5.

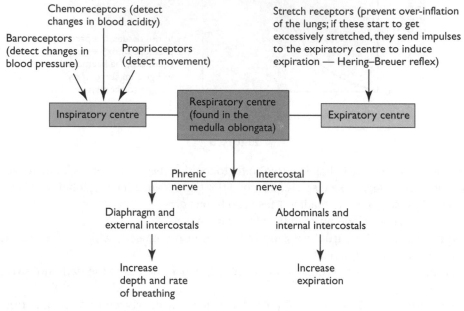

Figure 5

After studying this topic, you should be able to:
- describe the mechanics of breathing at rest and during exercise
- identify the different lung volumes and capacities and interpret them from a spirometer trace giving values at rest and during exercise
- describe gaseous exchange at the alveoli and the muscles

- explain the principles of diffusion and the importance of partial pressures
- explain how exercise can have an effect on the dissociation of oxygen from haemoglobin at the tissues (Bohr shift)
- explain how breathing is controlled

The vascular system: transport of blood gases

Circulation

There are two types of circulation:
- **pulmonary** circulation takes deoxygenated blood from the heart to the lungs and returns oxygenated blood from the lungs to the heart
- **systemic** circulation carries oxygenated blood from the heart to the body tissues and returns deoxygenated blood from the body tissues to the heart

Blood vessels

The vascular system consists of five different types of blood vessel that carry the blood from the heart, distribute it around the body and return it to the heart.

Arteries carry blood away from the heart. Each heartbeat pushes blood through the arteries by a surge of pressure. The elastic arterial walls expand with each surge, which can be felt as a pulse in the arteries near the surface of the skin. The arteries then branch off and divide into smaller vessels called **arterioles**, which in turn divide into microscopic vessels called **capillaries**. A capillary wall consists of a single layer of endothelium cells. Capillaries are only wide enough to allow red blood cells to pass through one at a time. The exchange of substances with the tissues takes place across the capillary walls and the blood then flows from the capillaries to the **venules**, which gradually increase in size and eventually form **veins**. To summarise, the order in which the blood flows through the vascular system is:

heart → arteries → arterioles → capillaries → venules → veins → heart

The important features of arteries, capillaries and veins are summarised in Table 6.

Table 6

Feature	Artery	Capillary	Vein
Tunica externa (outer layer)	Provides flexible support that prevents collapse under increased pressure	Absent	Thinner than in an artery
Tunica media (middle layer)	Thick with many elastic fibres	Absent	Thinner and less elastic than in an artery
Tunica interna (inner layer)	Smooth lining	Makes up the entire wall of the capillary	Smooth lining with valves to ensure blood flows in one direction
Size of lumen	Small	Microscopic	Large

Knowledge check 8

Give one structural feature of veins and one structural feature of arteries.

The pulse

The pulse is a wave of pressure generated when the left ventricle pumps blood into the aorta, which is the main artery. The pulse can be felt at a number of places in the body — the radial artery in the wrist and the carotid artery in the neck are the two most common sites. Other sites include the femoral, brachial and temporal arteries.

Venous return

This is the term used for blood that is returned to the right side of the heart through the veins. Up to 70% of the total blood volume is contained in the veins at rest. This provides a large reservoir of blood that can be returned rapidly to the heart when needed.

The heart can only pump out as much blood as it receives, so cardiac output is dependent on venous return. A rapid increase in venous return enables a significant increase in stroke volume and therefore cardiac output. Veins have a large lumen and offer little resistance to blood flow. By the time blood enters the veins, blood pressure is low. This means that active mechanisms are needed to ensure venous return:

- **Skeletal muscle pump** — when muscles contract and relax, they change shape so that the muscles press on nearby veins, causing a pumping effect and squeezing the blood towards the heart.
- **Respiratory pump** — when muscles contract and relax during inspiration and expiration, pressure changes occur in the thoracic and abdominal cavities, compressing the nearby veins and enabling blood to return to the heart.
- **Valves** — ensure that blood in the veins flows in only one direction: once the blood has passed through a valve, the valve closes to prevent the blood from flowing back.
- **Smooth muscle** — a thin layer of smooth muscle in the walls of the veins helps to squeeze blood back towards the heart.

Oxygen and carbon dioxide in the vascular system

Oxygen plays a major role in energy production. A reduction in the amount of oxygen in the body has a detrimental impact on performance. During exercise, when oxygen diffuses into the capillaries supplying the skeletal muscles, 3% dissolves in plasma and 97% combines with haemoglobin to form oxyhaemoglobin. At the tissues, oxygen dissociates from haemoglobin because of the lower pressure of oxygen that exists there. In the muscle, oxygen is stored by **myoglobin**. This has a high affinity for oxygen and stores the oxygen until it can be transported from the capillaries to the mitochondria. The mitochondria are the sites in the muscle where aerobic respiration takes place.

Carbon dioxide is transported around the body in the following ways:

- 70% is transported in the blood as hydrogen carbonate (bicarbonate) ions. The carbon dioxide produced by the muscles as a waste product diffuses into the bloodstream, where it combines with water to form carbonic acid. Carbonic acid is a weak acid that dissociates into hydrogen carbonate ions.
- 23% combines with haemoglobin to form carbaminohaemoglobin.
- 7% dissolves in plasma.

An increase in the level of carbon dioxide results in an increase in blood and tissue acidity. This is detected by chemoreceptors, which send impulses to the medulla. Heart rate, breathing rate and transport increase so that more carbon dioxide is exhaled and the arterial blood levels of both oxygen and carbon dioxide are maintained.

Blood pressure

Blood pressure is the force exerted by the blood against the blood vessel wall. It is measured at the brachial artery (in the upper arm) using a sphygmomanometer. A typical reading at rest is 120/80 mmHg (millimetres of mercury).

Knowledge check 9

How would performing a cool-down help venous return?

Knowledge check 10

How is carbon dioxide transported in the blood?

Blood pressure = blood flow × resistance

Blood pressure varies in the different types of blood vessel and is largely dependent on the distance of the blood vessel from the heart:
- arteries — high and in pulses
- arterioles — not quite as high as in arteries
- capillaries — pressure drops throughout the capillary network
- veins — low

Factors affecting blood pressure in blood vessels

The following factors can affect the pressure of blood in the blood vessels: contraction of the heart, stroke volume/cardiac output, blood flow, resistance, friction, elasticity, blood viscosity, lumen size, vasoconstriction, vasodilation and health factors such as diet, atherosclerosis, stress, age, level of fitness.

Blood velocity

The velocity of blood flow depends on the total cross-sectional area of the blood vessel. The smaller the cross-sectional area, the faster the blood flows. Although the capillaries are the smallest of the blood vessels, the fact that there are so many of them means that the total cross-sectional area is much greater than that of the arteries. This means that the flow of blood is slower in the capillaries and this allows enough time for efficient exchange of substances with the tissues. The relationship between blood velocity and cross-sectional area of the different blood vessels is shown in Figure 6.

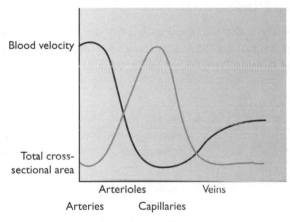

Figure 6

Effects of exercise on blood pressure and blood volume

During aerobic exercise, systolic pressure increases due to an increase in cardiac output. Diastolic pressure remains constant. During isometric work, diastolic pressure also increases due to increased resistance in the blood vessels.

A decrease in blood volume occurs during exercise when plasma moves out of the capillaries and into the surrounding tissues. After a period of training, blood volume increases, due mainly to an increase in the volume of blood plasma and a small increase in the number of red blood cells.

Examiner tip
Questions on blood pressure usually ask for an average reading, e.g. 120/80, and to identify what happens to blood pressure during exercise.

The vascular shunt

The distribution of blood flow is different at rest compared to exercise. During exercise, the skeletal muscles require more oxygen so more blood needs to be redirected to them in order to meet this increase in oxygen demand. The redirecting of blood flow to the areas where it is most needed is known as shunting or the vascular shunt mechanism.

This redirection of blood flow to the working muscles means that sports performers should ensure they do not eat less than an hour before competition. A full gut would result in more blood being directed to the stomach instead of the working muscles and this would have an effect on performance as less oxygen is being made available. Blood flow to the brain must remain constant as the brain requires oxygen to ensure brain function is maintained.

The control of blood flow

The **vasomotor centre** is located in the medulla oblongata of the brain. It controls both blood pressure and blood flow. During exercise, an increase in carbon dioxide is detected by chemoreceptors, while higher blood pressure is detected by baroreceptors. These receptors stimulate the vasomotor centre, which redistributes blood flow by **vasodilation** and **vasoconstriction**:
- Vasodilation increases blood flow.
- Vasoconstriction decreases blood flow.

Pre-capillary sphincters also aid blood redistribution. These are tiny rings of muscle located at the opening of capillaries. When they contract, blood flow is restricted through the capillary and when they relax, blood flow is increased.

Summary

After studying this topic, you should be able to:
- explain pulmonary and systemic circulation related to the various blood vessels (arteries/arterioles/capillaries/venules and veins)
- describe the venous return mechanisms
- understand how blood is redistributed during exercise (vascular shunt)
- describe how oxygen and carbon dioxide are transported in the blood (to include an understanding of the role of haemoglobin and myoglobin)
- explain what is meant by blood pressure and velocity and relate these terms to specific blood vessels

Cardiac function

The cardiac cycle

diastole the relaxation phase
systole the contraction phase

The diastole phase is when the chambers of the heart are relaxing and filling with blood. The systole phase is when the heart contracts and forces blood either around the heart or out of the heart to the lungs and the body. The diastole phase lasts for about 0.5 seconds; the systole phase lasts for 0.3 seconds. The cardiac cycle is summarised in Table 7.

Table 7

Stage	Action	Result
Atrial systole	Atrial walls contract	Blood is forced through the bicuspid and tricuspid valves into the ventricles
Atrial diastole	Atrial walls relax	Blood enters the right atrium via the vena cava and the left atrium via the pulmonary vein but cannot pass into the ventricles, because the tricuspid and bicuspid valves are closed
Ventricular systole	Ventricular walls contract	Pressure of blood opens the semilunar valves and blood is ejected into the pulmonary artery and the aorta. The tricuspid and bicuspid valves close
Ventricular diastole	Ventricular walls relax	Blood enters from the atria (passive ventricular filling, *not* due to atrial contraction). The semilunar valves are closed

The cardiac cycle is triggered by an electrical impulse called the cardiac impulse or the conduction system.

The conduction system

When the heart beats, blood flows through it in a controlled manner — in through the atria and out through the ventricles. Heart muscle is described as **myogenic** because the beat starts in the heart muscle itself, with an electrical signal in the sinoatrial node (pacemaker). This electrical signal then spreads through the heart in what is often described as a wave of excitation.

From the sinoatrial node (SAN), the electrical signal spreads through the walls of the atria, causing them to contract and force blood into the ventricles. The signal then passes through the atrioventricular node (AVN) in the atrioventricular septum. This delays the transmission of the cardiac impulse for approximately 0.1 seconds to enable the atria to contract fully before ventricular contraction begins. The electrical signal then passes down through specialised fibres called the bundle of His. This is located in the septum separating the two ventricles. The bundle of His branches into two bundle branches and then moves into smaller bundles called Purkinje fibres, which spread throughout the ventricles. When the impulse passes through these fibres, it causes them to contract.

> **Examiner tip**
> Remember the order:
> SAN › atrial systole → AVN → bundle of His → bundle branches → Purkinje fibres→ ventricular systole

Cardiac terms

Stroke volume

This is the amount of blood pumped out by the left ventricle in each contraction. The average resting stroke volume is approximately 70 ml. Stroke volume is determined by:
- Venous return — the volume of blood returning to the heart through the veins. If venous return increases, stroke volume will also increase (i.e. if more blood enters the heart, more blood is pumped out).

- The elasticity of cardiac fibres — the volume of blood in the ventricle increases during diastole and stretches the cardiac fibres. The more they stretch, the greater the force of contraction, which increases ejection fraction. This is called **Starling's law**.
- The contractility of the cardiac tissue (myocardium) — the greater the contractility of cardiac tissue, the greater the force of contraction. This results in an increase in stroke volume.
- An increase in the ejection fraction (the percentage of blood pumped out by the left ventricle per beat). An average value is 60% but it can increase by up to 85% following a period of training.

Heart rate

This is the number of times the heart beats per minute. The average resting heart rate is approximately 72 beats per minute.

Cardiac output

This is the amount of blood pumped out by **each** ventricle per minute. It is equal to stroke volume multiplied by heart rate:

cardiac output (Q) = stroke volume × heart rate

$$Q = 70 \times 72$$
$$= 5040\,ml\ (5.04\ litres)$$

Cardiac output and exercise

Regular aerobic training results in hypertrophy of the cardiac muscle — the heart muscle gets bigger. This has important effects on stroke volume and heart rate, and therefore on cardiac output. A bigger heart enables more blood to be pumped out per beat (i.e. stroke volume increases). In more complex language, the end diastolic volume of the ventricle increases. If the ventricle can contract with more force and push out more blood, the heart does not have to beat so often. Therefore, the resting heart rate decreases. This is called **bradycardia**. The increase in stroke volume and decrease in resting heart rate mean that cardiac output at rest remains unchanged. However, during exercise an increase in heart rate, coupled with an increase in stroke volume, results in an increase in maximum cardiac output.

Table 8 shows the differences in cardiac output (to the nearest litre) in a trained and an untrained individual at rest and during exercise. The individuals are aged 18 so their maximum heart rate is 202 beats per minute. (A person's maximum heart rate is calculated as 220 minus his/her age.)

Table 8

Condition	Stroke volume/cm³	Heart rate/bpm	Q/litres
Untrained, at rest	70	72	5
Untrained, during exercise	120	202	24
Trained, at rest	85	60	5
Trained, during exercise	170	202	34

This increase in maximum cardiac output has huge benefits for trained individuals. It means that more blood, and therefore more oxygen, is delivered to the working muscles. In addition, when the body starts to exercise, the distribution of blood flow changes — a higher proportion of blood passes to the working muscles and less goes to other organs such as the intestine.

Stroke volume in response to exercise

Stroke volume increases with exercise intensity but only up to 40–60% of maximum effort, at which point it levels out. One explanation is that the increased heart rate at near maximum effort results in a shorter diastolic phase. The ventricles have less time to fill with blood, so they cannot pump as much out.

Heart rate range in response to exercise

The heart rate response to maximal and submaximal exercise and during recovery from exercise is shown in Figure 7.

Figure 7

Key to the graphs:

a = **anticipatory rise** due to the action of the hormone adrenaline, which makes the heart beat faster and stronger

b = sharp rise in heart rate at the beginning of exercise, mainly due to anaerobic work

c = heart rate continuing to rise due to maximal workloads stressing the anaerobic system

d = 'steady state' as the athlete is able to meet the oxygen demand for the activity

e = rapid decline in heart rate as soon as the exercise stops, owing to a decrease in the demand for oxygen by the working muscles

f = slow recovery as the body systems return to resting levels (but the heart rate stays elevated to rid the body of waste products such as lactic acid)

Control of heart rate

Heart rate increases during exercise to ensure that the working muscles receive more oxygen. The heart generates its own impulses from the sinoatrial node but the rate at which these impulses are fired is controlled by two main mechanisms — neural and hormonal.

Examiner tip

If a question asks for the effects of a period of training on resting cardiac output, remember that cardiac output remains the same at rest. It is *maximum* cardiac output that increases.

Examiner tip

Past exam questions have asked about 'anticipatory rise' and 'steady state', so make sure you understand these terms.

Neural control involves the autonomic nervous system, which comprises the sympathetic system and the parasympathetic system. The sympathetic system stimulates the heart to beat faster; the parasympathetic system returns the heart rate to its resting level. The cardiac control centre located in the medulla oblongata of the brain coordinates these two systems.

The cardiac control centre is stimulated by:
- chemoreceptors — which detect increases in carbon dioxide and lactic acid and decreases in oxygen
- baroreceptors — which detect increases in blood pressure
- proprioceptors — which detect increases in muscle movement

Knowledge check 12

Explain how the increasing level of carbon dioxide in the blood raises heart rate.

The cardiac control centre then sends an impulse through the sympathetic nervous system or the cardiac accelerator nerve to the sinoatrial node and heart rate increases.

The **hormonal control mechanism** involves adrenaline and noradrenaline. These are stress hormones released by the adrenal glands. Exercise causes a stress-induced adrenaline response. This results in:
- stimulation of the sinoatrial node, which results in an increase in both the speed and force of contraction
- an increase in blood pressure due to the constriction of blood vessels
- an increase in blood glucose levels — glucose is used by the muscles for energy

Cardiovascular drift

It used to be thought that exercising at a steady level led to the body reaching a steady state where the heart rate remained constant. However, new research has shown that heart rate increases slowly. This is called **cardiovascular drift**. Cardiovascular drift is characterised by a progressive decrease in stroke volume and arterial blood pressure, together with the progressive rise in heart rate. It occurs during prolonged exercise in a warm environment despite the intensity of the exercise remaining the same. It is suggested that cardiovascular drift occurs because a portion of the fluid volume lost when we sweat comes from the plasma volume. The decrease in plasma volume reduces venous return and stroke volume. Heart rate increases to compensate and maintain constant cardiac output. To minimise cardiovascular drift, it is important to maintain high fluid consumption before and during prolonged exercise.

Effects of training on the heart

Physiological adaptations take place after a period of training and these will make the initial training sessions appear very easy. This is because more oxygen can be taken in, transported and utilised by the muscle cells.

athlete's heart common term for an enlarged heart caused by repeated strenuous exercise

hypertrophy increase in volume (organ gets bigger and stronger)

bradycardia a decrease in resting heart rate, usually below 60 beats per minute

The effects of training on cardiac function include athlete's heart, which is the common term for an enlarged heart caused by repeated strenuous exercise. Due to the increased demands of exercise, the chambers of the heart enlarge, as does muscle mass (hypertrophy). This results in an increase in the volume of blood that can be pumped out per beat and per minute, i.e. a rise in stroke volume and maximum cardiac output. Consequently, the heart has to contract less frequently and there is a decrease in resting heart rate (bradycardia).

Increased capillarisation of the heart muscle increases the efficiency of oxygen diffusion into the myocardium. Resistance or strength training causes an increase in the force of heart contractions due to a thickening of the ventricular myocardium. This increases stroke volume and the ejection fraction, as a higher percentage of blood is pumped out of the heart.

Summary

After studying this topic, you should be able to:
- describe the stages of the cardiac cycle and link them to the conduction system
- give definitions of cardiac output, stroke volume and heart rate and explain the relationship between them
- understand Starling's law of the heart
- explain heart rate range in response to exercise and describe the hormonal and nervous effects on heart rate
- explain the role of blood carbon dioxide in changing heart rate
- explain cardiovascular drift
- describe the concept of cardiac hypertrophy and how it is linked to bradycardia and athlete's heart

Analysis of movement

AQA only examines shoulder and elbow action in push-ups, over-arm throwing and forehand racket strokes, and hip, knee and ankle action in running, kicking, jumping and squats.

Axes and planes of the body

To help explain movement, the body can be pictured as having a series of imaginary slices running through it. These are called **planes of movement**. They divide the body in three ways:
- The **sagittal** plane is a vertical plane that divides the body into right and left sides.
- The **frontal** (coronal) plane is also a vertical plane but this divides the body into front and back.
- The **transverse** plane is a horizontal plane that divides the body into upper and lower parts.

The body (or body parts) moves in one or more of these planes, depending on the action being performed. In a full twisting somersault, for example, the gymnast moves in all three planes.

There are three **axes of movement**:
- The transverse axis runs from side to side across the body.
- The sagittal axis runs from front to back.
- The vertical axis runs from top to bottom.

Most movements occurring at joints are related to both axes and planes. For example, flexion and extension occur in a sagittal plane about a transverse axis; rotation occurs in a transverse plane about a vertical axis; abduction and adduction occur in a frontal plane about a sagittal axis.

Examiner tip
All movements at the ankle, knee and hip in the run, jump, kick and squat occur in a sagittal plane about a transverse axis.

Analysis of movement

AQA will only ask questions on seven sporting actions and these require particular movements. For each of these sporting actions, you do not need to learn all the movements the joints are capable of. These are summarised in Tables 9 and 10.

Table 9 Ball-and-socket joints

Joint	Articulating bones	Movement	Agonist
Hip	Pelvis and femur	Flexion Extension	Iliopsoas (hip flexors) Gluteus maximus
Shoulder	Scapula and humerus	Flexion Extension Horizontal flexion (adduction) Horizontal extension (adduction)	Anterior deltoid Latissimus dorsi Pectoralis major Latissimus dorsi

Table 10 Hinge joints

Joint	Articulating bones	Movement	Agonist
Elbow	Radius, ulna and humerus	Flexion Extension	Biceps brachii Triceps brachii
Knee	Femur and tibia	Flexion Extension	Hamstrings Quadriceps
Ankle	Tibia, fibula and talus	Plantarflexion Dorsiflexion	Gastrocnemius Tibialis anterior

Practical examples

Right leg action in kicking

This is illustrated in Figure 8.

- Hip joint — flexion
  - agonist: hip flexors (iliopsoas)
  - antagonist: gluteus maximus
- Knee joint — extension
  - agonist: quadriceps (rectus femoris)
  - antagonist: hamstrings (biceps femoris)

Figure 8

Leg action in squats (downward phase)

This is illustrated in Figure 9.

- Hip joint — flexion
  - agonist: gluteals
  - antagonist: iliopsoas
- Knee joint — flexion
  - agonist: quadriceps
  - antagonist: hamstrings

In these two joints, the agonist and antagonist appear to be the wrong way around. This is because an eccentric contraction is being performed during the downward phase.

Figure 9

Forehand racket stroke

This is illustrated in Figure 10.

- Shoulder from a to c — horizontal flexion (adduction)
  - agonist: pectoralis major
  - antagonist: latissimus dorsi
- Elbow from c to d — flexion
  - agonist: biceps brachii
  - antagonist: triceps brachii

Figure 10

Types of muscular contraction

A muscle can contract in three different ways, depending on the muscle action that is required.

Concentric contraction

The muscle shortens under tension — for example, during the upward phase of an arm curl, the biceps brachii performs a concentric contraction as it shortens to produce flexion of the elbow.

Eccentric contraction

Examiner tip
In the seven sporting actions examined by AQA, eccentric contractions only take place in the downward phase of a squat and a push-up.

The muscle lengthens under tension (and does not relax). When a muscle contracts eccentrically, it is acting as a brake to help control the movement of the body part during negative work. For example, when landing from a standing jump, the quadriceps muscles are performing negative work as they are supporting the weight of the body during landing. The knee joint is in the flexed position but the quadriceps muscles are unable to relax, as the weight of the body ensures that they lengthen under tension.

Isometric contraction

Examiner tip
A question that requires an isometric contraction for the answer will normally include the words 'still', 'stationary' or 'held'.

The muscle contracts without lengthening or shortening. The result is that no movement occurs. An isometric contraction occurs when a muscle acts as a fixator or against a resistance.

Muscle function

A muscle can perform two functions:
- **agonist** — the muscle shortens under tension to produce movement
- **antagonist** — the muscle relaxes or lengthens to allow the agonist to shorten

Antagonistic muscle action

Examiner tip
Be careful: sometimes the agonist does not automatically become the antagonist when the movement changes. In the downward phase of the press-up, the tricep is still the agonist since it is now lengthening as it contracts in order to control the lowering of the body as it performs an eccentric contraction.

Using flexion of the elbow as an example, the biceps brachii contracts and is responsible for the movement. It is said to be acting as an agonist or prime mover. An antagonist muscle is one that works in opposition to the agonist. When the biceps brachii is contracting, the triceps brachii is lengthening and acting as the antagonist. When one muscle is acting as an agonist and the other is acting as the antagonist, the muscles are said to be working together as a pair to produce the required movement. This is called **antagonistic muscle action**.

Levers

A lever has three main components:
- a pivot (fulcrum)
- the weight to be moved (resistance)
- a source of energy (effort or force)

In the body, the skeleton forms a system of levers that allows us to move. The bones act as the levers, the joints are the fulcrums and the muscles provide the effort.

The main functions of a lever are:
- to increase the speed at which the body can move
- to increase the resistance that a given effort can move

Classification of levers

There are three types of lever:

- First-order lever — the fulcrum is between the effort and the resistance. First-order levers can increase both the effects of the effort and the speed of the body. An example can be seen in the elbow during extension of the arm.
- Second-order lever — the resistance lies between the fulcrum and the effort. Second-order levers generally increase only the effect of the effort. Plantarflexion of the ankle involves the use of a second-order lever.
- Third-order lever — the effort lies between the fulcrum and the resistance. Third-order levers are responsible for most of the movements of the human body. They can increase the body's ability to move quickly but in terms of applying force they are very inefficient. An example can be seen in the forearm during flexion of the elbow.

The **effort arm** or **force arm** is the shortest perpendicular distance between the fulcrum and the application of force (effort). The **resistance arm** is the shortest perpendicular distance between the fulcrum and the resistance. Figure 11 illustrates the force arm and the resistance arm in a third-order lever.

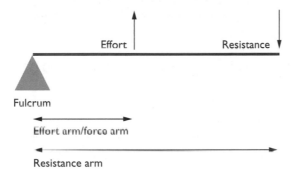

Figure 11

When the resistance arm is longer than the force arm, the lever system is at a **mechanical disadvantage**. This means that it cannot move as heavy a load but it can move the load faster. When the force arm is longer than the resistance arm, the lever system is at a **mechanical advantage**. This means that it can move a large load over a short distance and requires little effort.

Examiner tip

AQA only asks you to analyse five joints. They are all third-order levers except for the ankle, which is a second-order lever, and extension of the elbow joint, which is a first-order lever.

Knowledge check 13

Name and sketch the lever system that operates during extension of the elbow.

After studying this topic, you should be able to analyse the required sporting actions through knowledge of the following:

- the type of joint, articulating bones, joint actions, main agonists and antagonists, and the types of muscle contraction (concentric, eccentric and isometric) related to these sporting actions

- relate the movements occurring at joints to planes and axes
- identify the three classes of lever and give examples of their use in the body
- explain the relationship of levers to effective performance, with reference to mechanical advantages and disadvantages, and range and speed of movement

Summary

Applied exercise physiology in practical situations

This section will be taught through the practical component of your course (Unit 2). It will be examined as part of the extended question in Section B of the Unit 1 test.

Principles of training

An effective training programme will include the five principles of training:

- **specificity** — the training should be relevant
- **progression** — this involves the gradual application of overload
- **overload** (**FITT**) — this is achieved by increasing one or more of the following:
  - **frequency** (the number of times that you train per week)
  - **intensity** (how hard you work)
  - **time** (the length of the training session)
  - **type** of training
- **reversibility** — this is often referred to as detraining
- **tedium** — tedium has to be avoided, so a training programme needs to have variety to help maintain interest and motivation

Calculating working intensities for optimal gains

Heart rate

Heart rate training zones can be used to gauge how hard you are working. Most training zones are calculated from maximum heart rate, which is calculated as 220 minus age. So if you are 17, your maximum heart rate is 220 – 17 = 203.

You need to work at a certain percentage of your maximum heart rate. The **Karvonen principle** is more accurate than other methods because it takes into account an individual's fitness level by using resting heart rate to work out the training zone. Karvonen suggests a training intensity of 60–75% of maximum heart rate, using the following calculation:

60% = resting heart rate + 0.60 × (maximum heart rate – resting heart rate)

75% = resting heart rate + 0.75 × (maximum heart rate – resting heart rate)

For a 17-year-old with a resting heart rate of 60 beats per minute, the calculation is:

60% = 60 + 0.6 (203 – 60)	75% = 60 + 0.75 (203 – 60)
= 60 + 0.6 × 143	= 60 + 0.75 × 143
= 60 + 86 = **146**	= 60 + 107 = **167**

So a 17-year-old with a resting heart rate of 60 beats per minute, working at an intensity of 60–75% of maximum heart rate, should be working with a heart rate between 146 and 167 beats per minute.

Borg scale

The Borg scale is a simple method of rating perceived exertion (RPE) and is used to measure a performer's level of intensity during training. Perceived exertion is how hard you feel your body is working. During exercise, the Borg scale is used to assign numbers to how you feel. If you feel you are working too hard, you can reduce the intensity. The most common RPE scales are the 15-point scale and the 9-point scale.

1 rep max (1RM)

When weight training, you need to work out your one repetition maximum (1RM) for each exercise, so that you can decide on the intensity that you want to train at. There are different types of strength and you need to decide which type you want to improve. Depending on strength type, you need to work at a certain percentage of your 1RM. For example:

- maximum strength, 85% and over of 1RM
- power (elastic strength), 70–85% of 1RM
- muscular endurance, 50–70% of 1RM

Fitness testing

Fitness testing measures a performer's ability. It can highlight strengths and weaknesses, motivate the performer and progress can be monitored through retesting. Table 11 shows the testing methods that can be applied to the different types of fitness.

Examiner tip
You need to be able to identify a fitness test for each type of fitness.

Table 11

Component	Method of testing
Cardiorespiratory endurance (stamina)	Douglas bag Multi-stage fitness test Step test
Maximum strength Explosive strength Static strength	Hand grip dynamometer 1RM (one repetition maximum) test *No stand-alone test*
Muscular endurance	NCF abdominal curl
Flexibility 1. Static 2. Dynamic	Sit-and-reach test Shoulder flexibility test
Speed	30 m sprint test
Power	Vertical jump
Coordination	Alternate hand/wall ball toss
Reaction time	Metre ruler test
Balance	Balance board
Agility	Illinois agility run

Validity and reliability of testing

When carrying out the various fitness tests, it is important to consider their validity and reliability.

Validity — does the test measure exactly what it sets out to? For example, the 'sit-and-reach' test for flexibility only covers the hamstrings and lower back. Therefore it is a valid test for the lower body but not for the upper body.

Is the test sport specific? It is important to conduct a test that replicates sporting actions and uses the muscles in the same way they are used in the performer's activity. For example, the multistage fitness test involves running, so it is valid for a games player where a lot of running is involved, but less so for a cyclist or a swimmer.

Reliability — is the test accurate? In order for the step test to be reliable, the correct procedure must be maintained, i.e. everyone who completes the test should do so at the same rate, height and cadence and there should be full extension between steps.

When testing, the following factors should be taken into account:
- The tester should be experienced.
- The equipment should be standardised.
- Sequencing of tests is important.
- Performers should be motivated to complete the test to the best of their abilities.
- Tests should be repeated to minimise the effects of human error.

Examiner tip

Make sure you can relate validity and reliability to each test for each fitness component.

Principles of maximal and submaximal tests

Maximal tests are performed when the athlete is working at maximum effort, usually to exhaustion. The tests are reliable and objective. Examples of anaerobic maximal tests are the 30 metres sprint and the Wingate test. Aerobic maximal tests include the multistage fitness test and Cooper's 12-minute run.

Disadvantages of these types of tests are as follows:
- It is difficult to ensure that the performer is actually working to a maximum.
- It is hard to stay motivated when pushing yourself to exhaustion.
- There are possible dangers of over-exertion and injury.

Submaximal tests are not exhaustive — they do not require the performer to work at maximal levels. Aerobic examples of these tests include the Harvard step test and the PWC170 test. Motivation is not an issue but these tests rely on data that are predictive or estimated, so there are problems with accuracy and objectivity.

Warming up and cooling down

The warm-up

Warming up prepares the body for exercise and should be carried out at the start of every training session. The first stage of a warm-up should be light cardiovascular exercise, such as jogging, to gently increase the pulse. This increases cardiac output and breathing rate, and directs more blood to the working muscles via the vascular shunt.

The second stage involves stretching and flexibility exercises, especially with the joints and muscles that will be most active during the training session.

The third stage should include the movement patterns to be carried out — for example practising shooting in basketball and netball, or dribbling in hockey and football.

These three stages together increase the amount of oxygen delivered to the muscles and at the same time reduce the risk of injury.

A warm-up has the following physiological effects:
- The release of adrenaline increases heart rate and dilates the capillaries, allowing more oxygen to be delivered to the working muscles.
- Muscle temperature increases, which enables oxygen to dissociate more easily from haemoglobin and allows for an increase in enzyme activity, making energy readily available.
- The speed of nerve impulse conduction increases, which raises alertness.
- The increase in muscle temperature leads to greater elasticity of the muscle fibres, which increases the speed and force of muscle contraction.
- Efficient movement at joints occurs through an increased production of synovial fluid.

The psychological benefits of a warm-up include:
- It enables the performer to focus on the task in hand.
- It reduces anxiety.
- It allows mental rehearsal.

The cool-down

A cool-down should be performed after any physical activity, as it helps to return the body to its pre-exercise state more quickly.

A cool-down consists of light exercise to keep the heart rate elevated. This keeps blood flow high and allows oxygen to be flushed through the muscles, oxidising and removing any lactic acid that remains. Performing light exercise also allows the skeletal muscle pump to keep working, which maintains venous return and prevents blood from pooling in the veins.

A cool-down may help to limit the effect of DOMS, which arises from structural damage to muscle fibres and connective tissue surrounding the fibres, usually following excessive eccentric contraction when the muscle fibres are put under a lot of strain.

The psychological value of a cool-down includes:
- It allows the performer to focus on errors before the next game.
- It reduces stress.

Principles of safe practice

Apart from warming up and cooling down to help prevent injury and muscle soreness following exercise, there are some other factors to consider:
- Which exercises to perform and in what order — e.g. in circuit training the muscle groups should be rotated.
- Dehydration — performers should drink plenty of water during exercise.
- Rest days or recovery periods should be included in training sessions.
- The correct techniques must be used, especially in stretching and weight training.

DOMS delayed onset of muscle soreness, which usually occurs 24–48 hours after exercise

Examiner tip
Make sure you can both explain how to carry out a warm-up/cool-down and give the physiological reasons why we perform them.

- Equipment must be safety-checked.
- Athletes training in a cold environment should wear plenty of layers of clothing.
- Sports halls should be clean and free from potential dangers.
- Differences in performance due to gender and age should be considered. Men generally have more strength than women but the opposite can be true for flexibility.
- Training should be progressive, whether you are fully fit or returning from injury.

Training methods

Continuous training

This involves exercise without rest intervals, which places stress on the aerobic energy system. It concentrates on developing endurance. Examples include cycling, jogging and swimming. To make improvements in aerobic fitness, it is important to apply the principles of training (see page 30):

- Train at least three times per week.
- Train at 60–75% of maximum heart rate, as outlined earlier (Karvonen principle, page 30).
- Train for at least 20 minutes but ideally between 30 minutes and 2 hours, to ensure the aerobic system is working fully.
- Apply the principle of overload — after a few weeks your body will adapt to the exercise and resting heart rate will decrease, so to ensure you are working at 60–75% of maximum heart rate, you will have to work harder by increasing frequency, intensity or time.
- Training should be specific to the requirements of the activity (it has been suggested that training should be over a distance of 2–5 times that covered in the activity).
- Do not overdo it.
- Keep training interesting by varying the training loads, skills and activities.
- Your level of aerobic fitness will drop if you stop training.

Fartlek training

This is a slightly different method of continuous training. The word 'fartlek' means 'speed-play'. The pace of the run is varied to stress both the aerobic and the anaerobic energy systems. Fartlek is much more demanding and will improve an individual's VO_2(max) and recovery. A typical session lasts for 40 minutes, the intensity ranging from low to high.

Interval (intermittent) training

Interval training can be used to improve both aerobic and anaerobic capacities. It involves periods of work interspersed with recovery periods. Four main variables are used to ensure the training is specific:

- the duration of the work interval
- the intensity or speed of the work interval
- the duration of the recovery period
- the number of work intervals and recovery periods

Interval training can be adapted to overload each of the three energy systems. Anaerobic intervals should be short distance, high intensity; aerobic intervals should be long distance, submaximal intensity (see Table 12).

AQA AS Physical Education

Table 12

Energy system	Duration/ distance of work interval	Intensity of work interval	Duration of recovery	Number of work intervals/ recovery periods
ATP–PC	10s/60m	High	30s	10
Lactic acid	35s/200m	High	110s	8
Aerobic	6min/1500m	Submaximal	5min	3

Strength training

Improvements in strength result from working against a resistance. The training programme should be specific to the needs of the activity. The following factors must be considered:
- the type of strength to be developed — maximum, power (elastic) or muscular endurance
- the muscle groups to be improved
- the type of muscle contraction performed in the activity — concentric, eccentric or isometric

Strength training can also be used to increase muscle growth. In this case, any exercises performed must overload the anaerobic energy systems, which will result in hypertrophy of fast-twitch fibres.

Strength can be improved by doing the following types of training:
- weights — high weights for maximum and elastic strength, low weights for muscular endurance
- circuits for muscular endurance
- plyometrics and pulleys for elastic strength and power

Weights

Weight training exercises are usually described in terms of sets and repetitions. The number of sets and repetitions and the amount of weight lifted depend on the type of strength to be improved.

Before designing a programme, the maximum amount of weight that the performer can lift with one repetition must be found. Then, if maximum strength is the goal, high weights with low repetitions should be lifted, e.g. 2–6 reps at 80–100% maximum strength. If muscular endurance is the goal, more repetitions of lighter weights should be done, e.g. three sets of 10 reps at 50% maximum strength.

The exercises fall into four groups:
- shoulders and arms, e.g. bench press, curls, pull-downs
- trunk and back, e.g. sit-ups, back hyperextensions
- legs, e.g. squats, calf raises, leg press
- whole body exercises, e.g. power clean, snatch, dead lift

The choice of exercise should relate to the muscle groups used in sport — both the agonists and antagonists.

Circuit training

In circuit training, the athlete performs a series of exercises in succession. The exercises should include arm exercises (e.g. press-ups and triceps dips), leg exercises (e.g. squat thrusts) and trunk exercises (e.g. sit-ups and dorsal raises), as well as cardiovascular exercises such as jogging and skipping.

The athlete's body weight is used as resistance, and each exercise concentrates on a different muscle group. Circuits are usually designed for general body conditioning and are easily adapted to meet the needs of a particular activity.

Plyometrics

If leg strength is crucial to successful performance, for example in the long jump and 100m sprint in athletics, or rebounding in basketball, then plyometrics is a method of strength training that can be used to improve power or elastic strength. It works on the concept that muscles can generate more force if they have previously been stretched. In plyometrics, on landing, the muscle performs an eccentric contraction (lengthens under tension) followed immediately by a concentric contraction as the performer jumps up. This stimulates adaptations in the neuromuscular system and results in a more powerful concentric contraction of the muscle group being worked.

Mobility (flexibility) training

Mobility training aims to improve the stretch in the muscles and connective tissue. A stretch should be held for at least 30 seconds and a session should last for 10 minutes. With regular and repeated stretching, the soft tissue can elongate and this may be beneficial in avoiding injury. The three main types of flexibility training are:
- static stretching
- ballistic stretching
- PNF

Static stretching can be active or passive. In active stretching, the performer works on one joint, pushing it beyond its point of resistance, lengthening the muscles and connective tissue surrounding it. In passive stretching, the stretch occurs with the help of an external force, such as a partner, gravity or a wall.

Ballistic stretching involves performing a stretch with swinging or bouncing movements to push a body part even further. Only individuals who are extremely flexible, such as gymnasts and dancers, should perform this type of stretching.

PNF (proprioceptive neuromuscular facilitation) is where the muscle is contracted isometrically for a period of at least 10 seconds. It then relaxes and is stretched again, usually going further the second time.

Examiner tip

Make sure you can describe each of these training methods in detail and know which fitness component they are relevant for, e.g. continuous training improves stamina.

Summary

After studying this topic, you should be able to:
- apply your knowledge of the training principles to practical situations
- calculate working intensities in terms of heart rate and Borg scale
- understand the importance of a warm-up and cool-down

- identify the various methods of training
- give an explanation of fitness tests for specific fitness components
- understand the difference between validity and reliability, and apply these concepts to the various fitness tests

Skill acquisition

Characteristics of skill

Skilled performances are:
- **learned** — the performer has spent time practising the movement
- **efficient and economical** — the movement is performed quickly and easily, without wasting energy
- **goal-directed** — the performer has a predetermined result in mind
- **fluent** — the action is smooth and movements flow together
- **aesthetic** — the action is pleasing to watch
- **consistent** — the performer is able to repeat the action successfully time after time
- **technical** — the movement matches the demonstration shown

Examiner tip
Ensure you include the key words when you give a definition of skilled performer. Check how many marks are available — there might be more than 1 mark on offer. Use the mnemonic LEGFACT to help you.

Types of skill

The types of skill that are important in PE are:
- **motor** skills — involving movement and muscular control (e.g. performing a cartwheel)
- **cognitive** skills — involving thinking and thought processing (e.g. in badminton, a player thinks tactically and plays a long overhead clear to drive the opponent to the back of the court, followed by a drop shot)
- **perceptual** skills — involving the detection and interpretation of information (e.g. a goalkeeper in netball judges the flight of a lob pass coming into the circle and intercepts it)
- **psychomotor** skills — involving the processing of information quickly and putting decisions into action (e.g. in football, a defender sees an attacker about to make a run into space and reacts quickly to track back to block any passes to him/her)

Skill and ability

Abilities differ from skills. You need to know the differences between the two terms. Abilities are:
- **innate** — ability is genetically determined, whereas skill is learned
- **stable** and **long-lasting**, whereas skill can be developed and changes over time
- **foundations of skills** — you need ability to perform the skill

Performers need natural ability to reach the highest levels in sport. For example, top-level gymnasts are born with the ability of flexibility.

Knowledge check 14

Describe the terms 'skill' and 'ability'.

Types of abilities

There are two types of ability:
- **Gross motor abilities** involve physical movements. They relate to physical fitness and include speed, strength, stamina and suppleness/flexibility.
- **Perceptual** or **psychomotor abilities** involve sensing, interpreting and processing information — the ability to make a judgement and put it into action.

Classification of skills

A continuum is an imaginary sliding scale on which skills can be placed between two extremes to show a gradual increase or decrease in characteristic. Continua can be used to classify skills and to develop knowledge and understanding of the characteristics of skills. This is useful in structuring practices when taking on the role of leader or coach. Classification can help us to teach, practise and improve skills in the most efficient way.

Environmental influence

Skills are classified as **open** or **closed** depending on whether the surroundings change so that the performer has to use perception to make a judgement (see Figure 12).

Figure 12

Open skills are affected by the surrounding environment, which is constantly changing. The performer must adapt to these changes — for example, movements of team-mates and the opposition. The performer must use perception and make decisions. The skill is often externally paced.

Closed skills are not affected by the environment. They can be practised in a stable environment and therefore become habitual. The skill is usually self-paced and the performer rarely uses perception.

Continuity

The **continuity** continuum classifies skills as discrete, serial or continuous (see Figure 13).

Figure 13

Discrete skills have a distinct beginning and ending. The performer has to start the skill from the beginning to repeat it.

Serial skills are made up of a number of discrete elements, which are combined in a particular order to form a more continuous task. Each part can be practised separately.

Continuous skills have no distinct beginning or end. The skill is often cyclic. The end of one part of the movement becomes the beginning of the next.

Muscular involvement

Skills are classified as **gross** or **fine**, depending on the groups of muscles involved and the level of intricate, precise movement required (see Figure 14).

Figure 14

Gross skills involve movement of large muscle groups. Fine skills involve precise, intricate movements and accuracy using small muscle groups.

Pacing

The **pacing** continuum is based on who has control of the speed and timing of the skill during performance. If a movement is **self-paced**, the performer controls the timing, speed and rate of execution of the (usually closed) skill. If a movement is **externally paced**, the timing, speed and rate of the (often open) skill are determined by the environment (see Figure 15).

Figure 15

Example

A tennis serve is:

- closed, because the environment remains the same
- discrete, because it has a clear beginning and ending
- gross, because it is an explosive movement and several of the major muscle groups are used
- self-paced, because the speed and timing are controlled by the performer

---

After studying this topic, you should be able to:
- state the characteristics of skills and abilities, giving at least three for each (remember that 'smooth' and 'fluent' for skill counts as the same point, as does 'innate' and 'genetic' for ability)
- distinguish between skill and ability (this is a common question)

- define the various types of skills and abilities and give examples
- classify skills and justify this from your practical activities — explain *how* you reached your decision on where to place the skill on the continua

Summary

Information processing

Models of information processing

You need to understand both the Whiting and the Welford models of information processing. The models use slightly different terminology but the key processes are the same (see Figures 16 and 17).

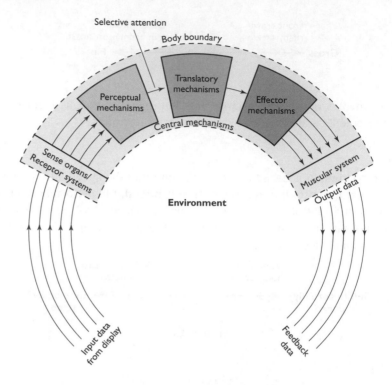

Figure 16 The Whiting model

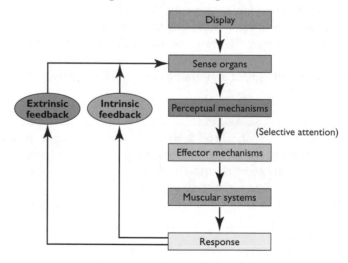

Figure 17 The Welford model

- The **display** and **input data** from the display. The display is the sporting environment and all the information contained in it. For example, the display for a rugby player includes the ball, team-mates, opponents, pitch markings, posts, the referee and linesmen, the crowd and the coach. Some of this information will be relevant to the performer and some will be irrelevant.

- **Sense organs** or **receptor systems**. Three senses are used to detect information from the display — vision (e.g. seeing the ball and opponents), audition (e.g. hearing the shouts from the coach concerning tactics, or the crowd calling 'man on') and proprioception, which tells us about the position of our bodies and what our muscles and joints are doing. Proprioception consists of **touch**, **kinaesthesis** and **equilibrium**. Kinaesthesis is the inner sense that tells us whether the movement is correct or not. Equilibrium gives information about whether the body is balanced.

- **Perceptual mechanism**. This interprets the information received by the sense organs. A decision on what action should be taken is made, sometimes with the help of previous experiences stored in the memory by using the DCR process. The relevant information (such as the ball, opponents and team-mates) is filtered from the irrelevant information (e.g. the crowd, linesmen etc.) by selective attention. Only the relevant information is acted upon; the irrelevant information is disregarded. For example, the rugby player sees a high ball and judges its speed travelling towards him. He compares it with stored memories and recognises that he has received a high ball before. Using selective attention, he focuses on the ball and disregards the crowd. He then decides on a plan of action or an appropriate response — he decides to turn sideways and jump to receive the high ball.

- **Translatory mechanism** (Whiting only). Using the information from the perceptual mechanism, the correct response is selected in the form of a motor programme.

- **Effector mechanism**. Once the plan of action is selected, the motor programme is put into action by sending impulses through the nervous system to the relevant working muscles, enabling them to carry out the movement.

- **Muscular system**. The muscles that are needed to jump and to catch the ball receive the impulses and are ready.

- **Response** or **output data**. The movement is performed.

- **Feedback** or **feedback data**. Once the motor programme has been put into action, information about the movement is received. This could be intrinsic (e.g. knowing that the ball was caught correctly because it 'feels' right, the ball is in my hands and I have landed on two feet so I feel balanced) or extrinsic (e.g. the coach shouts 'good jump, great catch' or the crowd cheers). This information can be used to assist future performances.

The memory system

The memory system is an integral part of information processing. It stores and retrieves information, makes comparisons with previous movement experiences and selects which motor programme to retrieve in order to produce the movement.

Three components make up the **multi-store model** and you need to understand the features of each.

DCR process Detection of environmental stimuli, **C**omparison with information stored in the memory and **R**ecognition of environmental stimuli

selective attention filtering the relevant from the irrelevant information

Knowledge check 16

What are the roles of the perceptual, translatory and effector mechanisms?

intrinsic feedback from within the performer using proprioception

extrinsic feedback from an outside source

Examiner tip

Ensure that you can define each part of both models and illustrate with a clear practical example.

Short-term sensory store

The features of the short-term sensory store (STSS) are as follows:

- *All* the information (relevant and irrelevant) is held briefly — for approximately 0.25–1 second.
- It has an unlimited capacity.
- The perceptual mechanism determines which information is relevant.
- Selective attention is operational. The relevant stimuli are attended to while the irrelevant stimuli are ignored. For example, a tennis player focuses on the ball when serving and disregards the crowd. This is important because it:
  - aids concentration
  - improves reaction time
  - filters out distractions
  - controls arousal levels
  - reduces the chance of information overload in the short-term memory
- Selective attention can be enhanced by:
  - practising with distractions and learning to block them out
  - making the stimuli more intense, e.g. using bright coloured bibs or equipment
  - the coach pointing out which stimuli to attend to
  - positively transferring skills (see pages 52–53) from one situation to another

Information from the STSS goes into the short-term memory.

Short-term memory

The short-term memory (STM) is known as the **working memory**. Its features are:

- Only relevant stimuli enter.
- Limited storage space of 7 ± 2 items.
- Information is stored for up to 30 seconds but this can be increased with practice.
- Information that is not rehearsed may be lost.
- It is responsible for executing the motor programme.
- Information is encoded and passed to the long-term memory.

Long-term memory

The features of the long-term memory (LTM) are as follows:

- Information enters the LTM through practice.
- Information can be stored permanently.
- It has unlimited capacity.
- Information is stored as motor programmes.

Strategies to improve retention and retrieval

A number of strategies can be applied to help store and remember information.

- **Practice** or **rehearsal** — repetition of a skill stores the motor programme in the LTM.
- **Linking/association/past experiences** — relating new information to that already stored. For example, when learning to serve in tennis, the performer might link it to the basic over-arm throw that he/she has experienced earlier (see positive transfer on page 53).

Knowledge check 17

Where in the model does selective attention occur?

Examiner tip

Remember to be specific — for example, instead of saying 'The STSS stores information for a small amount of time', be precise and state that it is 0.25–1 second.

Examiner tip

Do not confuse the STSS and the STM — this is a common mistake.

Knowledge check 18

List the features of the STM.

- **Chunking** — small pieces of information can be memorised together to extend the capacity of the STM. For example, instead of teaching a trampoline sequence as individual movements, the coach could 'chunk' three or four movements together. However, coaches should avoid giving too much information at one time because the STM can easily become overloaded.
- **Enjoyable/interesting/novel experiences** — if information is presented in a new or distinctive way, it is more likely to be remembered.
- Make it **meaningful** — if the learner understands the relevance of the skill to the performance, he/she is more likely to remember it.
- **Chaining** — information should be presented in an organised manner. For example, the elements of a tumble sequence in gymnastics should be presented in order to make it easier for the learner to remember.
- **Mental rehearsal/imagery** — visualising the skill or going over it in the mind will help the learner to remember what is needed to perform the skill. This is why demonstrations are important.
- **Reinforcement/rewards** — information is more likely to be remembered if the learner receives positive feedback or reinforcement, or is rewarded with praise after a correct response.

Reaction time

Definitions

Simple reaction time is when there is one stimulus and one response. Reaction time will be very short. For example, in a swimming race, the stimulus is the starter signal and the only response is to dive in.

Choice reaction time is when there are several stimuli and/or several possible responses. Reaction time will be slower. For example, in football several team-mates may be calling for a pass, and there may be several possible responses in terms of who to pass to and what type of pass.

reaction time + movement time = response time

Factors affecting reaction time

A number of factors affect reaction time. They include:
- **age** — reaction time increases (slows) with age
- **gender** — generally males have faster reaction times than females
- **stimulus intensity** — if the stimulus is bright (e.g. use of pink balls in cricket) or loud (e.g. a shout), it is easier to detect and reaction time will decrease
- **temperature** — the colder the body, the slower the reaction
- **previous experience** — experience of a skill speeds up reactions
- **anticipation** — predicting a movement correctly can reduce reaction time
- **drugs and alcohol** — drugs can speed reaction time up but alcohol slows it down
- **choices** — the more choices we are presented with, the slower we react (see Hick's law)

Knowledge check 19

Distinguish between simple reaction time and choice reaction time.

reaction time the time from the onset of the stimulus to the onset of the response

movement time the time from the onset of the task to the completion of the task

response time the time from the onset of the stimulus to the completion of the task

Knowledge check 20

Draw a diagram to illustrate the relationship between reaction, movement and response times.

Examiner tip

Listing the factors alone may not be enough to gain credit — you must explain the effect on reaction time. For example, stating 'gender' alone will not get the mark — you must specify that generally women react more slowly than men.

Hick's law

Hick's law describes the impact of choice reaction time on performance. It is illustrated in Figure 18.

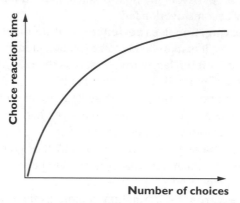

Figure 18

Strategies to improve the response time of a performer

There are a number of ways in which teachers and coaches can try to improve the response time of a performer. These include:
- practising responses to a stimulus (e.g. sprint starts to a gun)
- using mental rehearsal to help the performer focus on relevant information (selective attention)
- improving fitness levels
- warming up — making sure that the body and mind are prepared
- ensuring optimum arousal
- developing predictive skills — analysing the opponent's play in order to anticipate what he/she intends to do next

Psychological refractory period (PRP)

Anticipation can be:
- **temporal**, i.e. predicting *when* the action will be performed
- **spatial**, i.e. predicting *what* action will be performed

If we anticipate correctly, our response time will be quicker. However, if we anticipate incorrectly, our response time can be greatly increased. Figure 19 illustrates what happens if we anticipate incorrectly.

Figure 19

According to the **single channel hypothesis**, although we can pick up many stimuli at once, we can only *process* one piece of information at a time. If we are in the middle of processing one stimulus when a second stimulus arrives, it must wait until we have finished processing the first before it can be dealt with. This delay in processing causes our reaction time to increase and is known as the **psychological refractory period**.

We can use this in sport to try to slow down the opposition. For example, in rugby you are approaching your opponent with the ball in your hands. You feign a pass to the left. This is the first stimulus and the opponent begins to move in that direction. However, you decide to play a dummy and carry on running without releasing the pass. This is the second stimulus. According to the single channel hypothesis, the opponent has to process the first stimulus of the left pass before attending to the second stimulus.

Motor programmes

A motor programme comprises **subroutines**, which are the parts or mini skills that make up the whole skill. Motor programmes are formed by practice. When the skill becomes grooved or over-learned, the subroutines flow together and appear to be performed automatically. This occurs when the performer reaches the **autonomous** phase of learning (see page 47). Each time the motor programme is performed, it is modified and the adjustments are stored in the long-term memory.

The whole EMP is more important than the subroutines. The subroutines are **sequential** — that is, they are run in a specific order. Figure 20 shows an example of a motor programme.

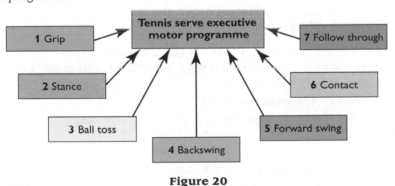

Figure 20

Knowledge check 21

What causes the delay known as the PRP?

Examiner tips

Ensure you can describe the PRP using a practical example. Do not confuse the PRP diagram with the Hick's law graph — this is a common mistake.

motor programme (or **executive motor programme**, **EMP**) a set of movements stored in the long-term memory that specify the components of a skill

Knowledge check 22

Draw a diagram to illustrate the EMP and key subroutines of a triple jump.

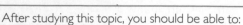

Summary

After studying this topic, you should be able to:
- draw Welford and Whiting's models and explain each component, using the same practical example to illustrate throughout
- describe the characteristics of each of the stores in the multi-store model of memory
- identify ways to improve the retrieval and storage of information and describe them
- describe the importance of selective attention to the STM (it filters the relevant information from the irrelevant and without it the STM would overload, as it has a limited capacity of 7 ± 2 items)
- define reaction time, movement time and response time using practical examples (use the sprint start because it is the easiest)

- draw and label a graph of Hick's law (this is usually worth 3 marks; to gain these marks you need to show an increase on the axes, label the axes and draw the curve correctly; an increase on the axes can be shown by using numbers, e.g. 1–9, or by putting arrows on the ends of the axes)
- describe the psychological refractory period (PRP) with a practical example (use the same example throughout — a dummy is easiest)
- identify and describe the factors affecting reaction time
- identify a motor programme and its relevant subroutines (these should be given in sequential order to ensure you gain credit)

Learning and performance

Stages of learning

The psychologists Fitts and Posner proposed the idea of three learning phases or stages, which relate directly to the acquisition of motor skills.

The cognitive phase

This is the first stage of learning. The key points are as follows:
- The learner begins to create a mental image of what the skill should look like.
- A demonstration may be necessary.
- Mental rehearsal of the skill is required.
- The performer has to consciously think about the skill and work out the main components.
- Trial and error is used to find the correct movement. Many mistakes are made.
- Movements might appear uncoordinated and jerky.
- The performer relies on extrinsic feedback from the coach to direct performance and highlight weaknesses. Feedback should be positive, so that the performer will persevere with the learning process.

For example, a hockey player who is learning to dribble is very slow to start with. Her movements are jerky and she often loses the ball because she hits it too hard. Her head is down and she watches the ball intently. She does not yet know how it is supposed to feel, so she relies on the coach for feedback. The coach gives demonstrations and the learner watches and works out each subroutine. She mentally rehearses dribbling constantly in this phase.

Examiner tip
If you are required to illustrate your answer with a practical example, to gain credit it must relate to the *same* characteristic that you have described.

Examiner tip
Do not confuse the cognitive phase with the cognitive theory of learning (see page 51). This is a common mistake.

The associative phase

This is the intermediate stage of learning — the longest phase as most performers remain in this phase.
- The performer must practise.
- Demonstrations, positive feedback and mental rehearsal are still required to aid learning.
- The performer becomes more proficient and makes fewer mistakes.
- Movements become smoother and more coordinated.
- The performer begins to focus attention on the finer aspects of the skill.
- Kinaesthesis begins to develop and intrinsic feedback can be used to correct movement.
- Knowledge of results and knowledge of performance are required.
- Motor programmes develop and are stored in the long-term memory.

For example, a gymnast on a beam practises and masters the basic skills, and is able to execute more complex movements. She can now use intrinsic feedback, and is becoming aware of how the movement should feel. She can look up and forward, rather than down at her feet.

The autonomous phase

This is the final stage of learning — the expert stage.
- Movements are fluent, efficient and habitual following extensive practice.
- Skills are executed automatically without consciously thinking about the subroutines.
- The performer can concentrate on the fine detail, tactics and advanced strategies.
- He/she uses intrinsic feedback to correct mistakes by means of kinaesthesis.
- Extrinsic feedback can be negative to aid error correction.
- Practice and mental rehearsal are important to stay at this level.

For example, a basketball player is able to dribble the ball fluently and consistently without having to look down at the ball. She is able to scan the court for passing options since the ball is controlled automatically. Errors are corrected immediately, without assistance from the coach.

Learning curves

A learning curve (Figure 21) illustrates the stages a performer goes through when learning a new closed skill.

Knowledge check 23

List three characteristics of each phase of learning.

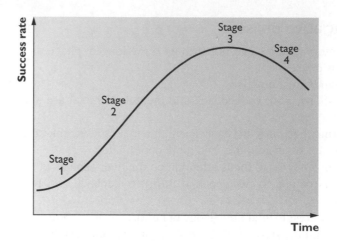

Figure 21

- Stage 1 — the performer is in the cognitive phase of learning, so the success rate is low. The performer is trying to work out the parts of the skill and is developing an understanding.
- Stage 2 — there is a sharp increase in success rate as the performer begins to grasp the skill. He/she enters the associative phase of learning and the skill begins to look more fluent. The performer's motivation levels are high as he/she is successful.
- Stage 3 — a plateau is reached where there is no improvement. Table 13 shows some causes of the learning plateau and solutions.
- Stage 4 — there is a dip in success rate. The performer lacks motivation and may experience drive reduction. A new task or challenge is required to remotivate the performer.

Table 13

Cause	Solution
Loss of motivation/boredom	• Set new tasks/challenges • Use variable practice • Offer tangible rewards
Mental/physical fatigue	• Allow performer to rest • Use distributed practice
Performer has reached ability limit	• Allow performer to compete against others of similar ability
Poor coaching	• Try a variety of coaching methods • Try an alternative coach
Incorrect goals set	• Set goals using the SMARTER principle (see page 53)

Motivation

Extrinsic motivation

Extrinsic motivation can be **tangible**, such as a trophy or medal, or **intangible**, such as praise from the coach.

Knowledge check 24

Sketch and fully label a diagram of a learning curve.

Examiner tip
You must be able to say why the plateau in learning occurs and offer a direct solution that relates to the reason why.

motivation the desire to succeed, an individual's drive that inspires him/her to perform in sport

Extrinsic reward is a valuable motivator for a beginner, but will eventually undermine intrinsic motivation. Withdrawing extrinsic rewards can lead to withdrawal from participation, especially with young performers.

Intrinsic motivation

Intrinsic motivation is the inner drive and self-satisfaction that comes from performing. It is longer-lasting than extrinsic motivation. However, it is difficult for some performers to generate enough intrinsic motivation to continue participating in an activity.

Intrinsic motivation is less relevant at elite levels of performance.

Motivational strategies

A range of strategies can be used to maintain drive.

For cognitive performers:
- Giving praise and positive reinforcement readily.
- Tangible, extrinsic rewards (e.g. certificates, medals, player of the match awards) will attract performers initially, and should be given periodically.
- Intangible extrinsic rewards (e.g. praise and positive reinforcement) will lead to increased confidence.
- The activity should be fun and enjoyable.
- Tasks should be easily achievable to ensure success.
- Positive role models or significant others can help to motivate.
- Highlighting personal improvement potential, e.g. in increase of health and fitness.
- Variable practice should be used.

For more advanced performers in the associative and autonomous stages:
- Giving praise and positive reinforcement readily.
- Generating intrinsic motivation through performance goals, for example beating a personal best.
- Setting new, challenging goals, just within the performer's reach.
- Performing with an audience present.
- Punishing lack of motivation.
- Using peer-group pressure.

extrinsic motivation
motivation from an external source

intrinsic motivation
motivation from within the performer

Examiner tip
A 2/3-mark question requiring an explanation of motivation would expect you to include a definition *and* details of the types of motivation.

Knowledge check 25
Compare extrinsic and intrinsic motivation.

After studying this topic, you should be able to:
- describe the characteristics of the three phases of learning (students often have difficulty describing the associative phase — make sure that the practical examples you give are clear and linked to a characteristic you have given)
- relate the phases of learning to feedback, guidance methods and practice methods with practical examples
- draw a learning curve and describe the four stages (make sure you can identify the causes of, and solutions for, the plateau)
- define motivation and distinguish between intrinsic and extrinsic motivation, with practical examples
- describe ways of motivating performers

Summary

Theories of learning

Operant conditioning

Connectionist or associationist theories state that learning occurs as a result of creating strong learning bonds. A learning bond is a link that connects the stimulus with the response (the **S–R bond**). The S–R bond is strengthened by **reinforcement**.

Operant conditioning is a major connectionist theory put forward by the psychologist B. F. Skinner. It suggests that an S–R bond can be created by manipulating the performer's response. A coach can accelerate the trial-and-error learning process by using strategies to:

- make the adoption of the correct response stronger
- make the neglect of the incorrect response stronger

Strategies to strengthen the S–R bond and promote adoption of the correct response include:

- allowing early success — by setting easy targets (this could include adapting the sporting environment to ensure a correct response)
- reinforcing the correct action by offering praise — if an action is not reinforced, it will not be repeated

Reinforcement

Positive **reinforcement** involves endorsing the performer's action when it is correct, so that the action is repeated in the future. For example, when a footballer defends a corner well, the coach offers praise in the hope that the action will be repeated in similar situations in the future.

Negative reinforcement involves the coach saying nothing when a correct action is shown, following a period of criticism about an incorrect performance. For example, a netball coach has been criticising the GA for missing shots. When the GA scores a goal, the coach says nothing. The GA recognises that she has not been criticised and repeats the correct shooting action.

Punishment is a method of reducing or eliminating undesirable actions. It can involve extra training, substitution, fines or a ban. For example, a player who drops the ball in rugby training is instructed to perform sit-ups, or a player is banned for a set period of time for constantly fouling the opposition.

Thorndike's laws

The psychologist Edward Thorndike proposed three laws to create and strengthen the S–R learning bond through the application of reinforcement.

- **Law of exercise** — the performer must practise in order to strengthen the S–R bond. If an action is not practised, the bond will weaken.
- **Law of effect** — when a correct action is shown, a satisfier such as praise should be given to strengthen the S–R bond. When an incorrect action is shown, an annoyer such as criticism should be given to weaken the S–R bond.
- **Law of readiness** — an S–R bond can only be created if the performer is mentally mature enough to understand and physically able to cope with the demands of the task.

S–R bond the relationship or link between the stimulus (S) and the response (R)

Operant conditioning uses reinforcement and rewards to ensure that the correct action is repeated.

reinforcement the process of strengthening an action or behaviour so that it will be repeated; it can be positive or negative

Examiner tip

Both positive and negative reinforcement aim to see positive actions being repeated, while punishment aims to get rid of negatives. Also, do not confuse negative reinforcement with negative feedback.

Knowledge check 26

Compare positive reinforcement with negative reinforcement.

Knowledge check 27

How would you use Thorndike's laws when learning the javelin throw?

Cognitive theories

Cognitive theories suggest that learning occurs by thinking about the task and developing a full understanding or insight.

Gestalt theory is the major cognitive theory. The key points are:

- Skills should be taught in their entirety rather than being broken down into subroutines — by using **whole learning**, the performer gains a greater understanding of the skill and develops kinaesthesis of the whole skill.
- Performers should think about what is required and consider the **intervening variables** (i.e. problems that can hinder performance).
- Performers should use **perception** to make a judgement and interpret the information available.
- Performers should use memory or **insight** of similar situations to help grasp the task, and use **previous experience** to help with the current task

Social learning theory

The psychologist Bandura believed that we learn most effectively by copying the actions of others. The theory of observational learning involves watching a demonstration and replicating the model. Table 14 shows the four important elements outlined by Bandura.

Table 14

Factor	Learner	Coach
Attention	Must focus and concentrate on the model	Can highlight the key areas of the skill
Retention	Must remember the image	Should give a clear, correct image so that it can be remembered
Motor reproduction	Must have the necessary physical and mental ability and skill to replicate the demonstration	Should make sure the performer is physically and mentally capable of performing the skill
Motivation	Must have the determination to learn	Can reward or praise the performer to create the drive to learn

Learners are more likely to copy:

- significant others — those they respect and admire, including family members, coaches, teachers, peers and role models in the media
- models with similar characteristics (e.g. age, gender)
- actions that are successful
- actions that are reinforced

Schmidt's schema theory

Schema theory suggests that the same skills can be used in different sports because the performer develops a set of 'generalised movements' that allow skills to be adapted to suit the situation. This is why some performers are capable in many sports. The schema has two parts.

Insight learning involves thinking through the entire learning process and developing an understanding of the whole skill.

Examiner tip
Do not confuse insight learning with observational learning — this is a common mistake.

Examiner tip
Use the mnemonic WIVPIPE to help you to remember the key concepts of this theory.

Observational learning involves watching and imitating the behaviour of significant others.

Examiner tip
Motor reproduction does not mean practising the movement — this is a common mistake.

Examiner tip
When asked to describe the key parts of the model, do not simply repeat the key term as it will not gain credit. For example, instead of stating 'Attention means paying attention', say 'Attention requires full focus on the action'. Use the mnemonic ARMM to help you to remember Bandura's four key processes.

Knowledge check 28
List the four key processes of Bandura's model.

- The **recall schema** stores information and initiates the movement — it takes place before the action.
- The **recognition schema** controls and evaluates the movement — it takes place during and after the action.

The performer's experience draws together information from four areas, or **memory items**:

- The **initial conditions** — the player gathers information from the environment, such as the position of other players. For example, a centre player in netball has the ball in her hands and is on the edge of the shooting circle. The GS is unmarked to her left. She remembers being in a similar situation both in training and in previous games.
- The **response specification** is based on the initial conditions. The player decides what movement to do. She decides to send a short, flat, fast pass to the GS, as she is quite near, before her defender recovers her position.
- The **sensory consequences** — the player gathers sensory information about the movement using intrinsic feedback or kinaesthesis. As she passes the ball, she feels her elbows bend and knows that as the ball left her hands it felt correct. She felt that placed enough power and height on the pass.
- The **response outcomes** gather information about the result of the movement. Was it successful or unsuccessful? For example, the GS received the pass and went on to score a goal.

Developing schemas

Coaches can organise practices to enable schemata to develop by:

- ensuring that practice is **varied** — to build a range of experience
- ensuring that practised skills are **transferable** from training to the game situation
- giving **feedback** to help improve skills
- giving **praise** and positive reinforcement
- **practising** a range of skills until they are well learned

Transfer of learning

Nearly all learning is based on some form of transfer.

- **Positive transfer** occurs when the learning of one skill facilitates the learning of another skill — for example, two skills that have a similar form: learning to throw in a rugby union line-out helps with long passing in American football.
- **Negative transfer** occurs when the learning of one skill inhibits the learning of an additional skill — for example, a netball player does not dribble when playing basketball because she transfers the static footwork rule across the two sports.
- **Proactive transfer** occurs when a previously learned skill has an effect on a skill learned later. It can be positive or negative. For example, learning to serve in volleyball now will (positively) affect the learning of a tennis serve in the future.
- **Retroactive transfer** occurs when new skills influence the learning and performance of a skill learned previously. This can also be positive or negative. For example, learning a golf drive may affect a hockey stroke (negatively) when you go back to playing hockey, because your swing is too high.

Knowledge check 29

List the two parts and four memory items of a schema.

Examiner tip

You must learn all parts of the schema theory and be able to apply it to a single practical situation. Do not change your practical example for each part.

Transfer explains the effect that the learning of one skill may have on the learning of another skill.

Examiner tip

When answering questions on transfer, you must describe the impact on sports skills (e.g. netball chest pass and basketball chest pass), not sports generally (e.g. netball and basketball). You must be able to give clear practical examples to illustrate your answers.

- **Bilateral transfer** is the transfer of skills from one side of the body to the opposite side. For example, learning how to perform snooker shots with one hand and then transferring to the other hand.
- **Zero transfer** occurs when there are no similarities between the tasks and therefore there is no effect on either skill. For example, learning to Eskimo roll in a canoe and learning an overhead clear in badminton will have no effect on each other.

To ensure positive transfer, the coach should:
- ensure that the performer's first skill is grooved
- highlight the potential for transfer
- ensure that the practice environment for both skills is similar
- make practice sessions as close to the game situation as possible
- give praise, reinforcement and rewards when positive transfer takes place as this will motivate the performer

To limit the effects of negative transfer, the coach should:
- ensure that the first skill is grooved before the second skill is presented
- highlight the differences in the skills, and therefore the potential for negative transfer
- ensure that the performer understands all the components of the skill

When a performer transfers learning from one skill to another, he/she builds a range of experiences and is able to adapt his/her motor programmes and performance to suit other environmental situations. An adapted motor programme is called a schema. Some performers appear to have a natural sporting ability, enabling them to be proficient in a number of skills and sports. They are *transferring* skills and using their experiences of other sports to help in the current situation.

Goal setting

Research has shown that setting goals has a positive effect on performance. The benefits of setting goals include:
- giving the performer an aim or focus
- increasing motivation
- increasing confidence levels
- controlling arousal levels
- focusing efforts in training and game situations

Types of goal

There are three types of goal:
- **Process goals** are set to improve technique.
- **Performance goals** are set to improve from previous attempts, e.g. personal bests.
- **Product** or **outcome goals** are based on winning.

Principles of goal setting

When setting goals, the SMARTER principle should be applied:
- **S**pecific — goals should be detailed and exact to target the weakness for the individual performer, for example reaching level 10.5 on the multi-stage fitness test.

Examiner tip
When describing positive/negative transfer, do not state 'has a positive/negative effect' as this is a repeat of the question and will not gain marks. You must be more precise.

Examiner tip
Remember that proactive transfer refers to the effect on new skills, while retroactive refers to old skills.

Knowledge check 30
List the six types of transfer.

Examiner tip
Be aware of the inextricable link between schema theory and transfer of learning.

- **M**easurable — goals must be quantifiable to track progress, for example making ten tackles in the next half.
- **A**greed — goals must be concurred by the performer and the coach so that they have shared responsibility for achieving the goal, for example you and your coach deciding to reduce your 400 m time by 2 seconds.
- **R**ealistic — goals have to be within the performer's reach to increase confidence, for example aiming to run your first 10 km in under 55 minutes.
- **T**ime phased — a set period must be stated in which the goal should be reached, to allow progression to be monitored and evaluated, for example performing a personal best time in the 100 m freestyle by the end of next month.
- **E**xciting — the goal has to be motivational, for example learning to do a somersault on the trampoline by next week.
- **R**ecorded — the progress has to be written down, to account for progress. For example, the coach should document the height of every high jump you make so that progress can be evaluated.

> **Knowledge check 31**
>
> What acronym is used when setting goals?

Summary

After studying this topic, you should be able to:
- describe the three theories of learning and explain how a performer learns a skill using each method
- state Thorndike's laws and explain how they strengthen the S–R bond, by using practical examples
- describe and give examples of positive and negative reinforcement
- identify the four memory items of a schema and explain them using a single practical example
- understand the link with varied and realistic practices in the development of schemata

- describe and give examples of the various types of transfer — make sure you give clear examples, particularly with proactive and retroactive transfer
- show knowledge of the importance of transfer in developing schemata
- explain the benefits of setting goals and the SMARTER principle — do not forget the practical examples
- discuss the types of goals — stick to one example throughout process, performance and product goals, to illustrate your knowledge

Skill acquisition in practical situations

Factors to consider when coaching

The style of teaching and the type of guidance offered can determine the success of a training session and greatly influence the motivation and enjoyment levels of the performer. When planning training sessions, the coach should consider:
- the experience level of the performers/what phase of learning they are in
- the fitness levels of the performers
- whether the task is dangerous
- the classification of the skills being taught in terms of environmental influence, pacing etc.
- the level of motivation of the performers
- the size of the group

> **Knowledge check 32**
>
> What factors regarding the group should you take into consideration before a training session?

Teaching styles

Command style

The command style of teaching is best used:
- in dangerous situations
- when time is limited
- with cognitive performers
- with large groups
- with a task that has one correct response
- when the learner is fully aware of what is required

Disadvantages of the command style are:
- it discourages creativity
- there is no differentiation in tasks for different abilities
- learners may become bored and demotivated

command style style of teaching where the coach instructs the group and is in full control — he/she makes *all* the decisions

Reciprocal style

The advantages of the reciprocal style of teaching are:
- increased contact and communication between group members
- it is useful with mixed ability groups
- all ability levels develop, either as 'coach' or learner
- feedback is given instantly as there may be several 'coaches'
- coaches may develop new ideas

Disadvantages of the reciprocal style include:
- it is time-consuming
- student coaches may lack experience
- student coaches may instruct or demonstrate incorrectly

reciprocal style style of teaching where the coach delegates some of the teaching to the more able members of the group

Problem solving or discovery style

Advantages of the problem solving or discovery style of teaching include:
- increased contact and communication between group members
- it is useful with mixed ability groups
- it is motivational, since learners achieve at their own level
- creativity is encouraged

Disadvantages of the problem solving or discovery style are:
- it is time-consuming
- incorrect techniques can be developed
- it is difficult to give feedback to large groups
- there are safety implications of allowing learners to work independently

problem solving or discovery style style of teaching that involves the coach posing an open task for the learners to work through, discovering how to solve the problem in their own way in their own time

Methods of presenting practice

To decide on the best method of presenting a skill to the learner, the coach first has to consider the classification and organisation of the movement. The best practice method will allow the skill to become grooved or over-learned.

Knowledge check 33

Give two advantages and two disadvantages of each teaching style.

Whole practice

Whole practice is the best method for skills that are highly organised and cannot easily be broken down into separate subroutines. Examples include continuous skills, such as cycling and jogging, and simple, discrete skills where a single action is required, such as a forward roll.

- Whenever possible, skills should be taught as a whole, to develop the correct feel of the skill (kinaesthesis).
- It saves time in that there is no assembling of the parts.
- The performer gains a clear mental image of the whole skill, which can easily be transferred into real game situations.
- It is the best method for ballistic actions that cannot be broken down, for example a golf swing.
- It is the best method for performers in the autonomous phase of learning.

Part practice

The part practice method is best for skills that are low in organisation and easily broken down into subroutines. It is also useful for serial skills, as each of the discrete elements can be practised independently.

- It is good for cognitive learners because just part of the skill can be focused on, reducing the chance of overload.
- It can reduce fatigue in physically demanding skills. For example, the correct leg kick in front crawl could be the focus of teaching rather than the entire skill.
- It is useful when the task is dangerous.
- It allows the performer to build confidence and increases motivation.
- It aids understanding of complex tasks, since the skill is broken down.

Progressive part method

The progressive part method (sometimes called '**chaining**') attempts to solve one of the problems of part practice by maintaining the links between subroutines. The first subroutine or part of the skill is taught and practised until perfect. The other parts are then added sequentially until the whole skill can be performed. Progressive part practice is useful when teaching the main components of the triple jump, for example (see Figure 22).

Figure 22

Whole–part–whole practice

This method involves performing the whole skill and identifying any weaknesses. The weaker parts are practised in isolation and then integrated back into the whole skill. It is useful for learners performing complex tasks and for more experienced performers who may be encountering problems. For example, when teaching front crawl:

- The whole skill is introduced initially.
- The arm action is practised in isolation with the aid of floats.
- The whole skill is practised again with improved arm action.

Types of practice

Variable practice

Variable practice is best for open skills (see page 38). An example is changing from partner work to unopposed practice to three-versus-two in rugby — the players can therefore develop their passing techniques and positional skills, which can be transferred directly into a game situation. Benefits of variable practice include:
- Performers learn to respond to the changing environment.
- Decision-making and perceptual skills develop.
- Adaptations are stored and therefore the experience of the performer is expanded.
- It improves selective attention.

variable practice practice where the environment and/or skill is constantly changing

Massed practice

Massed practice is a useful method for improving discrete, closed or simple skills. The continuous aspect of this method helps to groove or over-learn skills so that they become habitual. It can be physically demanding, so is most effective with highly motivated or autonomous performers. A high level of fitness is essential, although it may be used to develop fitness in lower-level performers. Examples include a badminton player trying to perfect a short serve, and a trampolinist continuously practising a seat drop to make it habitual.

massed practice continuous practice without rest periods

Knowledge check 34
Distinguish between massed and distributed practice.

Distributed practice

In distributed practice, the physical practice time is often less than the rest period. This method is regarded as more effective than massed practice. It is useful for practising continuous, dangerous, complex or tiring skills. The breaks in performance allow for physical recovery, so it is useful for performers who lack physical fitness. The rest periods allow time for mental practice. Distributed practice can also be used with cognitive performers, the coach giving feedback during the rest periods. An example of distributed practice is a steeplechaser running laps of a running track followed by a rest period, during which he/she mentally rehearses the performance — seeing the stride pattern, clearing the barriers and the water barrier.

distributed practice practice with rest periods included

Examiner tip
Defining the practice types alone is not enough. Suggest which type of practice is best for different levels of performers, situations and skill types.

Mental practice

Mental practice has been found to improve reaction times and confidence and may increase motivation. The best improvements in performance are made when physical practice is combined with mental rehearsal.

Mental practice involves the performer going over the task in his/her mind without moving.

Methods of guidance

There are four types of guidance that can be used to help the learning process.

Verbal guidance:
- is often used in conjunction with visual guidance
- is useful for more advanced performers in the autonomous stage of learning
- can be given during a performance

Verbal guidance involves the coach instructing the performers in the key points of the skill — telling them what to do and how to do it.

- is useful for open skills, where the performer needs to make decisions and adapt quickly
- can be used to give tactical, strategic or technical information that a cognitive performer may not understand
- requires that information should be kept brief and meaningful to avoid overload

Visual guidance:
- could be a demonstration by the coach, a video, a skill card or a coaching manual
- is effective for performers in the cognitive stage of learning
- helps to build a clear mental picture of how the skill should be performed
- is a guidance where the performer can grasp the key components of the movement as his/her attention is focused
- is a guidance where the coach can change or modify the display — for example, placing a chalked square on a tennis court for the performer to aim for while practising serves

Both **manual guidance** and **mechanical guidance**:
- are effective for performers in the cognitive stage
- are useful in dangerous tasks as they improve safety
- reduce fear and anxiety and therefore build confidence
- allow the whole skill to be attempted
- allow the performer to develop kinaesthesis

The drawbacks include:
- The performer may become reliant on the support/aid.
- Incorrect kinaesthesis could develop.
- Bad habits might be instilled.
- The performer might become demotivated by feeling that he/she is not performing the skill alone.
- The physical contact or proximity of the coach may make the performer feel uncomfortable (manual only).

Types of feedback

Feedback plays a vital role in correcting errors and improving performance. There are several different types of feedback you need to be aware of. These are summarised in Tables 15–18.

Table 15

Intrinsic feedback	Extrinsic feedback
Comes from within (e.g. proprioceptors and kinaesthesis)	Comes from external sources (e.g. coach, team-mates, crowd)
Concerns the feel of the movement (e.g. the feeling of balance during a headstand)	Received via sight and hearing
Begins to develop in the associative phase of learning	Cognitive performers rely on extrinsic feedback since they haven't yet developed kinaesthesis
Autonomous performers use it to correct errors	Importance of developing intrinsic feedback should be highlighted to cognitive performers

Examiner tip

Defining the guidance methods alone is not enough. Ensure that you suggest which type of guidance is best for different levels of performers, situations and skill types.

Visual guidance involves the performer *seeing* the correct method of performing the skill.

Knowledge check 35

Distinguish between verbal and visual guidance.

Manual guidance involves the coach holding and physically 'shaping' the body to give the learner an idea of how the skill should feel.

Mechanical guidance involves the use of a piece of equipment or a device to aid and shape movement.

Knowledge check 36

Distinguish between manual and mechanical guidance.

feedback the information received about the skill by the performer during the course of a movement, or as a result of it

Table 16

Positive feedback	Negative feedback
Received when the movement is correct, to reinforce the action	Received when the movement is incorrect, to stop the incorrect action from being repeated
Can be intrinsic or extrinsic	Can be intrinsic or extrinsic
Used to motivate performers	Reduces the chance of bad habits developing
Essential for cognitive performers (e.g. a coach praising a novice hurdler for a quick trail leg action)	Used with more advanced performers who may begin to detect their own errors

Table 17

Knowledge of performance	Knowledge of results
Concerns the quality of the performance	Concerns the outcome of the performance
Technique-based — tells you *why* the movement was correct or incorrect	Results-based — was the movement successful or unsuccessful?
Can be intrinsic or extrinsic	Can be positive or negative
Used by experienced performers as they use kinaesthesis	Important for cognitive performers

Table 18

Concurrent	Terminal	Delayed
Continuous feedback received during the movement	Feedback received when the movement has finished	Feedback given at a later date
Can be intrinsic (kinaesthesis) or extrinsic (the coach giving instructions as you perform)	Extrinsic	Extrinsic
Autonomous	Cognitive/autonomous	Autonomous

Knowledge check 37

List the types of feedback available to a performer.

Examiner tip

Ensure you can link the type of feedback to the performer's phase of learning.

Summary

After studying this topic, you should be able to:
- identify the factors to consider before leading or coaching a practical session
- describe the various teaching styles and suggest advantages and disadvantages for each
- describe the various methods of practice and relate them to the skill classification
- link the methods of practice to the three phases of learning
- give advantages and disadvantages of each of the methods of practice and support your answers with practical examples (relate these to performer, situation and skill type)
- give advantages and disadvantages of each of the types of guidance and support your answer with practical examples (relate these to performer, situation and skill type)
- explain the various types of feedback, with examples, and relate them to the phases of learning
- discuss the benefits and functions of feedback

Opportunities for participation

Concepts

This section introduces some of the concepts, categorisations and benefits of physical activity to individuals and society. The key characteristics are features that help identify a particular concept. The objectives are the aims or functions of a concept for individuals or society in general.

Leisure time

Key characteristics

Leisure can be defined as spare time during which individuals can choose what to do. When all duties and obligations have been completed, there may be a little time left to spend as you wish. Some people like to relax and spend their free time inactively, while others look for excitement and danger — it is a matter of personal choice.

Key objectives

Functions of leisure for an individual can be summarised by a number of 's' words:
- **s**tress relief — relaxation, improve health and fitness
- **s**ocial benefits — meeting people, forming friendships
- physical **s**kill development
- **s**elf-confidence and **s**elf-fulfilment improvement

Leisure time used in a positive way also has a number of functions for society. It:
- civilises society (is a form of social control)
- encourages social and racial mixing, job creation etc.

Active leisure as physical recreation

Key characteristics

Recreation can be defined as the **active** aspect of leisure. It is entered into voluntarily during free time and people have a choice concerning which activities to take part in. The focus is on **participation** rather than results. It has a low level of organisation/structure.

Key objectives

Recreation provides many benefits for individuals, including the opportunity to:
- relax
- be creative
- socialise
- improve health and fitness

Recreation can also be said to increase conformity and morality in society as a whole. Social benefits of recreation include:

- community integration through mass participation events
- social control and crime reduction
- employment opportunities
- less strain on the NHS
- economic benefits

Play

Key characteristics

A useful way of remembering the key features of play is to use the mnemonic 'TESCO':
- **T**ime and space are flexible
- **E**njoyment
- **S**pontaneous
- **C**hild-like
- **O**ptional whether you play or not

Key functions of play

Play has many different functions both for adults and children.

The key feature of adult play is motive. For an adult, play has mainly psychological benefits as it can provide stress relief, an escape from the reality of everyday life and an opportunity to relax.

The main function of play for children is to **master reality**. Through play, children can learn:
- social skills, such as making friends and cooperation
- physical skills, such as coordination
- emotional skills, such as accepting defeat
- environmental skills, such as safety awareness
- cognitive skills, such as decision making
- moral skills, such as fair play

Comparing and contrasting play and recreation

Characteristics shared by play and recreation include the following:
- They are entered into of one's own free will.
- The primary motivation is enjoyment.
- They have an informal structure — for example, flexible rules and time.
- The outcome is non-serious and a casual attitude is adopted.

Differences between play and physical recreation include the following:
- While intrinsic enjoyment is the primary aim for both play and recreation, other motives are likely to be involved in the recreation process — adults may use recreation to escape the stresses of daily life, and view it as an opportunity to improve their health and wellbeing.
- While both play and recreation have a flexible, loose organisation or structure, recreation is slightly more organised than play.

Examiner tip

Make sure you can identify a number of different reasons why participation in active leisure is encouraged by local and central government.

Knowledge check 38

State the key reasons why local and central governments in the UK have developed policies to encourage physical activity.

Examiner tip

Questions are often set about key characteristics of a concept either in isolation (e.g. play) or in comparison (e.g. play and recreation).

Sport

Key characteristics

Sport is different from play and physical recreation in that it is competitive, strict rules apply and extrinsic rewards are available for winning. The more you can identify features such as competition, high skill levels and physical exertion, the more likely it is that the activity can be classified as sport.

Sport is:

- **s**erious/competitive — the aim is to win, with the 'win at all costs' attitude or sportsmanship
- **p**rowess — high skill levels, particularly by professionals and elite performers, commitment to train/improve
- **o**rganised — sport has strict rules and regulations, NGBs setting rules
- **r**ewards — available for winning (extrinsic) and intrinsic satisfaction
- **t**ime and space restrictions apply, as sport is far more structured and organised

Knowledge check 39

Identify three characteristics that distinguish sport from play.

Key functions

Sport serves a number of important functions for individuals, including:

- improved health and fitness
- increased self-esteem and self-confidence
- opportunities for socialising

Table 19 compares physical recreation and sport.

Examiner tip

Sport is often compared to concepts at the opposite end of the continuum (e.g. play).

Table 19

Physical recreation	Sport
Immediate pleasure	Sometimes enjoyable, particularly in victory, but may involve anxiety and pain
Participation provides intrinsic rewards and enjoyment	There may be extrinsic rewards
Length of participation is the individual's choice	Time constraints on training and length of game
Spontaneity exists	Less spontaneous because of game plans
Level of training is the individual's choice	Serious training is required
Flexible rules	Strict rules

Outdoor and adventurous activities

Outdoor and adventurous activities (OAA) form one of the six areas of National Curriculum PE (outdoor education) but are also important as outdoor recreation.

Characteristics of OAA as outdoor education

OAA as outdoor education can be defined as 'the achievement of educational objectives via guided and direct experiences in the natural environment'. For example, pupils who are up a mountain and being formally instructed in skills such as map reading and taking a compass bearing are taking part in outdoor and adventurous activity in PE.

Functions of OAA in the National Curriculum

OAA have many functions, including raising awareness of and respect for oneself, others, the natural environment and danger or risk. Risks should be perceived only (i.e. in a pupil's head) rather than real (actual danger).

Outdoor activities such as hill walking, caving and canoeing can give personal challenges to individuals, as well as teaching them how to work effectively with one another (teamwork, cooperation). They can provide opportunities to experience the responsibilities of leadership, such as making decisions that affect the rest of the group. Communication skills and an awareness of an individual's strengths and weaknesses may develop.

A sense of adventure and excitement is an important part of the outdoor experience.

Outdoor activities need to be specifically linked to the natural environment (e.g. mountain walking and rock climbing). Such activities as part of compulsory National Curriculum PE belong under the overall umbrella of PE, and so involve the same potential set of values (physical skills, health and fitness improvement, social and cognitive development).

Factors influencing a pupil's OAA experience

OAA in most schools tends to be of relatively low quality. A number of factors may negatively affect a pupil's OAA experience:

- If staff lack specialist qualifications, experience or motivation, the opportunities for a positive and meaningful experience will be reduced.
- Lessons do not allow much time for OAA.
- Access or transport to the natural environment is a problem for many schools.
- Money and resources — the expense of undertaking OAA may be too much for many schools and parents. Specialist equipment may not be readily available.
- Parents and teachers are likely to be deterred by the inherent risks of certain activities such as skiing and mountain climbing

Key characteristics of OAA as outdoor recreation

The characteristics and functions of physical recreation are defined and explained on page 60. The key distinguishing feature of outdoor recreation is that it takes place in the natural environment, for example climbing a mountain or canoeing down a fast-flowing river.

Key functions of OAA as outdoor recreation

Individuals who choose to participate in outdoor recreation activities do so to:

- improve health and fitness
- relieve stress and relax
- develop self-esteem and self-confidence (personal challenge)
- develop an appreciation of the natural environment
- develop cognitive skills and decision-making abilities
- develop social skills and work as a team
- develop survival skills

Knowledge check 40

What are the key benefits that individuals receive as a result of participating in OAA (e.g. youngsters as part of outdoor education)?

Examiner tip

It is important to be able to give a critical evaluation of a pupil's OAA experience in relation to the factors identified here, and to appreciate that in many schools it is taught in a limited manner due to such factors. For example, orienteering activities may be restricted to the school grounds.

Summary

After studying this topic, you should be able to:
- show understanding of the characteristics and objectives of a range of concepts — in isolation and compared to and contrasted with one other
- explain the benefits of sport and leisure to individuals as well as to society in general (this is sometimes linked to government or local authority provision)

Current provision for active leisure

You need to know the characteristics and aims of the public, private and voluntary sectors in relation to active leisure provision in the UK.

Public sector provision

The important features of public sector provision (e.g. leisure centres, swimming pools, public parks) include:
- facilities are open to all, non-exclusive
- run by local authorities and managed by local authority employees
- run as business operations, with the aim of breaking even
- trade on set prices according to pre-set budgets
- facilities and services are of adequate or improving standard

Aims

Central government sees the provision of facilities for sport and recreation as increasingly important in today's society because of health and obesity issues. By providing facilities and schemes to increase participation in physical activity, local authorities aim to:
- increase health and fitness of individuals and improve the health and wellbeing of the community
- increase social control and reduce crime in the community
- improve social integration
- provide for social needs, equal opportunities and social inclusion
- regenerate areas (this may link to national government policy)

Such aims need to be achieved within financial constraints. Local authorities are required to break even and to give taxpayers value for money.

Private sector provision

Private sector leisure provision, such as the David Lloyd health clubs, have the following characteristics:
- They are exclusive, with a selective clientele — elitist.
- They are privately owned or belong to registered companies.
- They trade on profit-and-loss accounts — the main aim is to make a profit.
- They are managed by owners or appointed employees.
- They offer a high-quality service and facilities (at a price!)

Membership of private fitness clubs has become increasingly attractive to the general public in our health-conscious society.

Knowledge check 41

Identify the main aim of public sector sport/ recreation provision.

Advantages of private fitness clubs are that individuals have more choice of where to go to improve their health and fitness, with such clubs offering high-quality facilities and service to encourage continued participation. Personal trainers may help individuals with low levels of fitness or self-motivation. However, such high-quality provision is too expensive for the majority, who rely instead on cheaper alternatives within the public and voluntary sectors. Sometimes individuals are deterred from private-sector participation because it is viewed as elitist and exclusively for the rich.

Aims

The key aims of private sector provision are to:
- make a profit
- increase membership numbers
- provide an exclusive, high-quality service for members

Voluntary sector provision

Voluntary sector sports clubs, such as local athletics, rugby and tennis clubs, are:
- run by members or committees on a voluntary basis (this reduces costs and overheads)
- sometimes owned by members on a trust or charity basis
- financed by membership fees, fund-raising etc.
- run on a profit-and-loss basis — making a profit is not an overriding concern

Aims

Key aims of voluntary sector leisure provision are to:
- provide for grass-roots sports participation
- increase club membership and performance levels
- provide opportunities for people to meet others with similar interests
- seek funds from sponsors and the lottery to develop playing opportunities and facilities

Best value

'Best value' is a key government policy requiring local authorities and other related organisations to provide the best value for money possible. It is the principle on which local authorities decide who should run a particular service — who can provide the highest quality service at the best possible price.

Best value involves finding out what the public want, trying to deliver a service to match these standards, then reviewing whether their targets have been met or not.

Knowledge check 42

Identify three key characteristics of private sector provision for active leisure.

Examiner tip

Exam questions require knowledge of how the public sector compares to the private sector in relation to characteristics and/or aims.

Knowledge check 43

What are the key characteristics and aims of the voluntary sector?

After studying this topic, you should be able to:
- know and understand:
  - the characteristics and goals of the public, private and voluntary sectors
  - the advantages and disadvantages of the public, private and voluntary sectors
  - the concept of 'best value' in relation to public sector provision for sport/recreation
- identify the key characteristics of a particular sector and compare the different sectors
- understand the changing relationship between the public and private sectors with regard to provision for active leisure

Summary

Increasing participation: the role of schools and national governing bodies

Historical, social and cultural factors

Key characteristics of rational recreation

rational recreation the post-industrial development of sport into a 'structured/ organised' format

The **'R' factor** is a useful mnemonic to help you remember the key characteristics of rational recreation as they all start with the letter 'r':

- **R**egular — e.g. Saturday afternoon football
- **R**ules — National Governing Bodies of sport were formed who codified/devised rules for the conduct of a sport (e.g. FA 1863); they were written and complex
- **R**oles — players developed position-specific roles, e.g. defenders
- **R**evolution link — e.g. urban revolution led to a lack of space available in cities, which meant purpose-built facilities had to be built in the 'small areas' available
- **R**eferees — officials enforced the newly developed rules

Examiner tip

While the historical development of sport is covered in far more detail at A2, it is important for PHED 1 that you are able to identify a number of key characteristics of rational recreation.

How nineteenth-century public schools assisted in the 'technical development' of rational recreation

Nineteenth-century public schools:
- developed rules
- began intra- and inter-school sport
- employed coaches and trained to improve
- introduced use of officials
- played in a set kit
- used tactics

Legacy of the nineteenth-century public schools

The National Curriculum for PE (see page 69) emphasises the importance of team games in developing qualities such as sportsmanship, teamwork and leadership in individuals. Learning how to be competitive is an important part of modern life. Respecting opponents and officials are key aims today, as they were in earlier times. Fair play and sportsmanship are seen as positive qualities that can be developed through PE at school. Improved decision-making and cognitive skills are also seen as important values resulting from involvement in team games.

Development of PE in elementary state schools

You need to understand the following key terms:
- **Objectives:** reasons why different syllabuses were introduced and what they were trying to achieve (*aims*).
- **Content:** *what* was being taught in a lesson.
- **Methodology:** *how* a lesson was taught (and at times by whom?)

The Model Course 1902

Colonel Fox of the War Office introduced the Model Course of Physical Training in 1902 (see Table 20). It had a military emphasis with no educational focus and did not cater for children's needs. Its intention of improving the health and fitness of the children was questionable. The exercises were mainly static and dull. It lasted for just 2 years.

Table 20

Objectives	Content	Methodology
• to improve fitness (for military service) • training in the handling of weapons • to improve discipline	• military drill • exercises in unison • weapon training	• command–response (e.g. 'Attention', 'Stand at ease', 'Marching, about turn') • group response, no individuality • in ranks

Examiner tip

Questions on the Model Course will link to the characteristics of military drill and/or the aims of military drill.

Knowledge check 44

Identify three key aims of the Model Course.

Early developments in physical training (1904 and 1909 syllabuses)

Dr George Newman was a key influence in the development of the physical training (PT) syllabuses. He was appointed as Chief Medical Officer to the Board of Education. As a doctor, he was interested in the health-giving effects of exercise (see Table 21).

Table 21

Objectives	Content	Methodology
• therapeutic effects of exercise, with emphasis on respiration, circulation and posture • obedience and discipline still important • enjoyment • alertness, decision making, control of mind over body	• Swedish in character, with recreational aspects to relieve the tedium and monotony of former drill-style lessons • dancing steps and simple games	• 1904: 109 tables of exercises for teachers to follow • 1909: reduced to 71 tables • still formal, in ranks, with marching and free-standing exercises • still group response to commands • a kinder approach by teachers, some freedom of choice for teachers

1919 syllabus

Table 22 summarises the 1919 syllabus.

Table 22

Objectives	Content	Methodology
• enjoyment and play for the under-7s • therapeutic work for the over-7s • age differentiation starting to appear in PT lessons	• the exercises performed were similar to those in 1909 syllabus • a special section of games for the under-7s was included • not less than half the lesson was spent on 'general activity exercises' — active free movement, including small games and dancing	• more freedom for teachers and pupils • less formal than previous PT syllabuses

1933 syllabus

The 1933 PT syllabus was seen as a watershed between the syllabuses of the past and the physical education of the future (see Table 23).

Examiner tip

It is important to be able to identify similarities and differences between early state school PT (e.g. 1904) and late-twentieth-century PE (e.g. National Curriculum PE — see page 69).

Table 23

Objectives	Content	Methodology
• physical fitness • therapeutic results • good physique and posture • development of mind and body (holistic development)	• athletics, gymnastics and games skills • group work	• still direct style for the majority of the lesson • some decentralised parts to the lesson • group work/tasks throughout • special PE clothing worn during lessons • many schools now had specialist facilities available (e.g. newly built gymnasiums)

Development of state PE in the 1950s

Moving and Growing was produced in 1952 by the Education Department as a guide for primary schools. Primary school teachers were not trained in physical education, so they needed guidance to plan and deliver it. The term 'physical education' had evolved, giving a different emphasis from the earlier 'physical training'.

Rudolf Laban influenced the development of state PE in the 1950s with his work on movement to music, educational dance and creativity. His work became highly influential in *Moving and Growing* (1952) and *Planning the Programme* (1954).

Table 24 summarises the objectives, content and methodology of PE in the 1950s.

Knowledge check 45

Identify the key characteristics of post-Second World War/1950s state PE.

Table 24

Objectives	Content	Methodology
• to develop physical, social and cognitive skills • variety of experiences in a fun atmosphere • increased involvement for everyone, at their own level of ability	• agility exercises, gymnastics, dance and games skills • swimming • movement to music	• child-centred and enjoyment orientated • progressive • teacher guidance rather than direction • problem solving, creative, exploratory, discovery • individual interpretation of tasks encouraged • using apparatus in lessons — ropes, bars, boxes, mats

The start of a 'recreational focus'

In the last decades of the twentieth century, radical changes were made to the physical activities in state schools. The Butler Education Act 1944 required local authorities to provide recreational sporting facilities in schools. This was a very different philosophy from the one held at the beginning of the twentieth century, which believed that the working classes had no need for recreation. The secondary school teacher was now fully trained and therefore no longer dependent on following a syllabus drawn up centrally. Physical education teachers were to experience 40 years of a decentralised system, where they had autonomy and were able to choose their own physical education programmes.

National Curriculum PE

By the end of the 1980s, the government wanted:
- more control of education
- more teacher accountability
- national standards for physical education
- a wider range of activities to be taught

The 1988 Education Reform Act led to the introduction of National Curriculum Physical Education, which applied to all state schools. This represented a return to a centralised approach towards education. All state schools now follow set guidelines for set subjects to teach, which are inspected by Ofsted.

PE was made compulsory for all 5–16-year-olds, reinforcing its importance. Through physical education, children should be able to:
- achieve physical competence (i.e. improve physical skills)
- improve self-confidence and knowledge of strengths and weaknesses
- perform in a range of activities, including those that encourage active leisure
- improve health and fitness
- become a 'critical performer' (i.e. children should be encouraged to observe and analyse physical activities in a knowledgeable way)
- learn how to plan, perform and evaluate
- improve cognitive skills and decision making
- improve social skills and leadership qualities

Critical performer

The National Curriculum aims to provide students with knowledge of roles in sport other than performer. Roles such as official, coach, spectator and leader encourage students to appreciate physical activities in different ways, and possibly to take on some of these roles at various stages of their lives.

Areas of activity

The current aims of PE are to offer a broad range of physical activities. Concentrating on one activity would not provide a balanced physical development. The National Curriculum classifications are:
- game
- athletics
- swimming
- gymnastics
- dance
- outdoor and adventurous activities

Schools cannot offer every sport available but there should be a balance of activities — team and individual, competitive and non-competitive — selected from the categories listed above.

Physical Education compulsory, formally taught sports in primary and secondary schools, with a high level of structure/pre-planning

Examiner tip
The characteristics of PE are sometimes compared in exam questions to other concepts such as sport, active leisure etc.

Knowledge check 16
What important objectives does NC PE aim to fulfil?

Examiner tip
Make sure you can identify the aims of NC PE and the roles it encourages children to develop.

Factors that influence PE and sport provision in schools

A pupil's experience of PE and sport at school can be positive or negative, depending on various factors in individual schools.

- Timetable restrictions. Schools sometimes reduce the amount of time allocated to PE due to the demands of other, more 'academic' subjects. PE may be marginalised, particularly at Key Stage 4 when the demands of GCSE examinations are high.
- Lack of funding or resources. Budgets may restrict the quality and breadth of a pupil's PE experience. For example, many schools find the funding of swimming and OAA particularly difficult. Transport for fixtures might also be deemed too expensive and could negatively affect inter-school sporting opportunities.
- Quality of staffing. PE teachers and external coaches vary in terms of qualifications and their degree of commitment to PE/school sport.
- Quality of facilities. The availability of specialist facilities for offering a range of PE and sport varies throughout the country.
- School–club links. Links between schools and clubs can positively influence PE and school sport, by improving a pupil's access to high-quality coaching and facilities.

As well as the core curriculum lessons, children are offered many other sporting experiences at school. Extra-curricular activities are optional activities offered in schools during lunchtime and after school. They offer recreational experiences as well as competitive fixtures. This is also called **school sport**, which should be differentiated from physical education. Physical education refers to the compulsory core lessons.

In the UK, physical education and school sport have traditionally been kept separate, as they are believed to serve different aims. However, there is now a growing belief that these two strands should be brought closer together and initiatives are taking place to try to achieve this. Examples include the Physical Education, School Sport and Club Links (PESSCL) strategy and sports college status being given to some schools.

Current government policies

PE, School Sport and Club Links strategy

PESSCL is a national strategy aimed at increasing the uptake of sporting opportunities by 5–16-year-olds so that 85% of them experience a minimum of 2 hours' high-quality PE and school sport each week.

Sports colleges

Sports colleges are an important initiative designed to raise standards in PE/sport. Their main aims include:

- providing high-quality PE/sport (sharing good practice)
- increasing performance standards of pupils
- helping meet government targets for PE/sport
- providing high-quality teaching/coaching/SSCos (School Sport Coordinators)

Club Links

A school–club link is an agreement between a school or school sport partnership and a community-based sports club to work together to:
- meet the needs of all young people who might want to get involved in their sport/club
- help young people to realise their ambitions in sport and dance by providing pathways for them to follow
- provide new and varied opportunities for people
- agree good standards of provision, putting in place quality controls to ensure that standards remain high

The main aim of the Club Links programme is to increase the number of children participating in sports clubs.

National governing bodies: increasing participation

National governing bodies (NGBs) are required to open their sport to all sections of society, including those at grass-roots participation levels. Ways of achieving increased participation include:
- developing policies linking to specific target groups (e.g. people with disabilities, ethnic minorities)
- training more sport-specific coaches to encourage participation
- developing mini-games and modified versions of their sports to encourage participation at all levels of ability (e.g. high 5 netball, short tennis)
- making facilities more accessible, affordable and attractive and targeting funds at grass-roots levels and inner-city schemes
- improving awareness of the sport through publicity, advertising and use of positive role models

NGBs and whole sport plans (WSPs)

NGBs develop WSPs to present to Sport England to illustrate how they propose to increase participation as well as provide progressive opportunities towards elite-level performance in the sport they are responsible for.

The purposes of a WSP for NGBs include:
- an increase in the number of accredited clubs within a sport
- an increase in participation/number of active members of clubs
- an increase in the number of qualified coaches/volunteers delivering the sport
- increased performance levels in international sports competitions
- more funding for the sport via Sport England funding awards
- establishment of partnerships (e.g. PESSCL/PESSYP)

Examiner tip

Exam questions will not require knowledge of a specific NGB WSP, so you simply need to understand the general purposes of a WSP as stated here.

Sport England

Sport England is a government-funded agency responsible for developing a world-class community sports system. It published a new strategy in June 2008, designed to get more people playing and enjoying sport.

Sport England has three clear outcomes:

- **grow** — increasing participation
- **sustain** — maintaining participation
- **excel** — developing talent support systems

To achieve such aims, Sport England has developed a number of schemes/initiatives, such as:

- SSCos/PESSCL
- Active Places
- Sporting Equals
- RAMP
- Gifted and Talented
- Sportsmark
- Step into Sport
- Sport Action Zones
- Funding WSPs
- Free Swimming
- Sport Unlimited

Examiner tip

It is important to be able to identify a variety of different schemes/ initiatives that Sport England has developed to deliver on its mission of 'Grow, sustain, excel'.

Sports Leaders UK

Sports Leaders UK provides the opportunity and motivation for people to make a meaningful contribution to their local community through nationally recognised sports leadership awards. Two examples are:

- The Junior Sports Leadership Award for 14–16-year-olds, taught mainly within the National Curriculum for PE at Key Stage 4. The award develops young people's skills in organising activities, planning, communicating and motivating.
- The Community Sports Leadership Award, designed for the 16+ age group and delivered by schools, colleges, youth clubs and sports centres.

The Youth Sport Trust

The Youth Sport Trust is the key organisation with responsibility for developing school sport. It works with a range of partners including Sport England and Sports Leaders UK. One of its programmes is TOP Sport, which is a Key Stage 2 initiative, with modified equipment suitable for this age group (7–11), as well as lesson plans for teachers linked to NCPE.

Examiner tip

For the Unit 1 exam, you do not need to know the structure of organisations, but it is important that you know how they work in partnership to raise participation levels.

The Youth Sport Trust believes in the power of sport to improve the lives of young people. It believes that all youngsters should:

- receive an introduction to PE and sport that links to their developmental needs
- be able to experience and enjoy PE and sport as a result of high-quality teaching, coaching, equipment and resources
- be able to progress along a structured pathway of sporting opportunities (e.g. TOP programmes and extracurricular sporting opportunities via SSCos, Junior Athlete Education, Gifted and Talented etc.)

- develop a sporting lifestyle and foundation for lifelong participation/leadership involvement via initiatives such as Step into Sport, UK School Sport Games and Sky Sports Living for Sport

The post-school gap

There is a big drop in participation when young people leave school — the 'post-school gap' — which has concerned the government and sporting institutions for many decades. Table 25 summarises the reasons for this and the possible solutions.

Table 25

Reasons for the post-school gap	Solutions
Physical education is no longer compulsory	Improve links between schools and clubs so that continued participation is more likely
Young adults have competing leisure interests	Develop knowledge about the need for a healthy lifestyle
Facilities are no longer as accessible or free to use	Offer concessionary rates to young people with a limited disposable income
Traditionally poor links between schools and clubs	Link youth sections at clubs to schools (e.g. share facilities, coaches)

Reasons for government emphasis on PE and school sport

The government believes in the power of PE and sport to improve and enrich people's quality of life, to raise their self-esteem and confidence levels, as well as to provide enjoyment to individuals in society.

Sport is seen as having an important role to play in building stronger, safer communities, strengthening the economy and developing the skills of local people. It also meets the needs of improving the health and fitness of individuals and society in general.

Summary

By the end of this section, you should be able to explain:
- the historical and social factors that have influenced current PE/sport provision (e.g. public schools)
- the development of state PE from the early twentieth century to post-Second World War
- the characteristics of National Curriculum PE (Key Stages 1–4) and its relevance to increasing participation
- the factors affecting school PE provision and the impact it has on a pupil's PE experience
- how school–club links are affecting schools and clubs in providing sport and recreation opportunities for young people
- a number of initiatives (e.g. PESSCL strategy, TOP programmes, SSCos, sports colleges, Active Sports) and organisations (e.g. Sport England, Sports Leaders UK, Youth Sport Trust, national governing bodies of sport), and how they are benefiting individuals and communities by raising participation levels

Barriers to participation

There are a number of key terms you need to understand when studying equal opportunities in sport and recreation. Three of these — prejudice, discrimination and stereotyping — are important reasons for inequality, both in the past and at present.

- **Prejudice** means to form an unfavourable opinion of an individual, often based on inadequate facts (e.g. lack of tolerance of people from a specific race or religion).
- **Discrimination** is the unfair treatment of a person, racial group or minority — an action based on prejudice.
- **Stereotyping** is making simplistic generalisations about a group that allows others to categorise them and treat them accordingly.

Knowledge check 47

Explain the term 'discrimination'.

In Unit 1, four groups are identified (women, ethnic minorities, people with disabilities and lower social classes) and their lack of participation in sport can be linked to a number of factors, including prejudice, discrimination and stereotyping.

Increasing participation in sport is helping to achieve an important aim for local and central government — to decrease exclusion (and therefore increase inclusion) in society. Local and national governments continue to invest resources in sport and recreation schemes to try to create a sense of worth in society in an effort to combat social exclusion.

- **Social exclusion** occurs when certain sections of society are left out of the mainstream; this can happen when people suffer from a range of linked problems (e.g. unemployment, low income and poor housing).
- **Inclusive sport** means that all people have the right to equal opportunities according to their particular needs.

The performance pyramid

The performance pyramid helps to focus discussions about participation.

- The **foundation** level — sometimes called the grass-roots stage of development — is an introduction to physical activity for young children. Basic movement skills and a positive attitude to physical activity are developed from an early age.
- The **participation** level has an emphasis on fun, socialising and formation of friendships. At school this may be through **extra-curricular** activities.
- The **performance** level refers to e.g. county or regional levels of performance, and individuals receive specialist coaching to improve their standard.
- A limited few reach the **excellence** level. Such elite performers strive to represent their country and are fully committed to their sport.

Examiner tip

The PHED 1 exam will focus on the lower levels of the pyramid when looking at initiatives to raise participation as a result of various barriers being experienced at foundation/ participation levels.

Sport and mass participation

The idea of mass participation in sport is that everyone should have the chance to take part in sport as often as they like and at whatever level they choose. However, the reality does not always match the 'Sport for All' principle of equal opportunities.

Target groups are sections of society identified by Sport England as needing special attention. The aim is to raise participation levels so that they have equality of sporting opportunity. Target groups include ethnic minorities, women, young people (16–24), the elderly, lower social-class groups and people with disabilities.

Under-representation of women in sport

A number of reasons can be given to explain the under-representation of women in sport:
- stereotypical myths (e.g. the belief that physical activity could damage fertility, or that women are not aggressive)
- less media coverage
- fewer role models
- fewer sponsorship opportunities
- lower prize money
- negative effects of school PE programmes (e.g. lack of choice, rules on kit)
- lack of time due to work and family responsibilities
- lack of disposable income
- fewer female coaches and officials

Solutions to gender inequalities

Women's representation in sport is still low in relation to their numbers in society but improvements are being made. Reasons include:
- greater social acceptance of women having jobs and financial independence
- increased media coverage of women's sport
- positive female role models to aspire to
- education to refute stereotypical myths
- more women qualified to coach or officiate in women's (and in some cases men's) sport
- more clubs for women to join and competitions to enter
- the Women's Sports Foundation (see **www.wsf.org.uk**) promotes the benefits of exercise for women and works with other organisations to develop campaigns and policies, such as Sports Coach UK and Women into High Performance Coaching

Examiner tip
Be prepared to give reasons for lower participation by a specified 'target group' (e.g. lack of participation by teenage girls/women) as well as to suggest possible solutions to such barriers.

Race and religion in sport

Britain is a multicultural, multiracial, egalitarian society. Equal opportunities to participate in sport should exist for all racial groups in society. Such equality is not a reality due to many factors, including racism.

You need to understand the following key terms:
- **ethnic groups** — people who have racial, religious or linguistic traits in common
- **racism** — a set of beliefs based on the assumption that races have distinct hereditary characteristics that give some races an intrinsic superiority over others; it may lead to physical or verbal abuse

Racism is illegal but it still exists in society (and therefore sport as a reflection of society) on the basis of colour, language or culture. Racism stems from prejudice linked with the power of one racial group over another. This leads to discrimination, or unfair treatment. For example, teachers might assign students to certain sports or positions on the basis of ascribed ethnic characteristics rather than interests and abilities.

Other causes of under-representation of certain ethnic groups in sports and physical recreation include:
- conflict with religious observances
- a higher value placed on education (less support from family for sports participation)

- racist abuse
- fewer role models (particularly as coaches and managers)
- lower self-esteem and fear of rejection

Possible solutions to racial disadvantage and discrimination include:
- training more ethnic minority sports teachers and coaches, and educating them on the effects of stereotyping
- ensuring there is single-sex provision for Muslim women
- publicising and punishing severely any racist abuse
- organising campaigns against racism in sport
- making more provision in PE programmes for different ethnic preferences, e.g. relaxing kit and showering rules to accommodate cultural norms

Knowledge check 48

Give three reasons why some ethnic minority groups have lower participation rates than others.

Under-representation of people with disabilities in sport

Generally, people with disabilities have a low level of participation in sport. Disability may be physical, sensory or mental in nature, with all of these potentially affecting participation in a negative way. Society continues to discriminate against, and impose barriers on, disabled people's participation in physical activity.

The key terms you need to know are:
- **inclusiveness** — the idea that all people should have their needs, abilities and aspirations recognised, understood and met within a supportive environment
- **integration** — able-bodied and disabled people taking part in the same activity at the same time
- **segregation** — people with disabilities participating separately among themselves

Integration versus segregation

For some disabled individuals, inclusiveness is best realised by integration, while for others segregation may be better.

Potentially, integration has a number of benefits for disabled individuals, such as increasing their self-esteem, breaking down negative stereotypes and helping them to feel more valued in society. However, integration can also affect people with disabilities in negative ways, including safety concerns that have to be addressed and lower self-esteem if they are continually unsuccessful.

Segregation may lead to positive outcomes for the disabled, such as increased success. The negative aspects of segregation include reinforcement of the notion that the disabled are different from the rest of society, which may make them feel less valued and excluded from the mainstream.

Solutions to under-representation of disabled people in sport

Table 26 shows some causes of under-representation of disabled people in sport and the possible solutions to counteract it.

Table 26

Cause	Solution
Negative self-image, lack confidence	Provide opportunities for success
Low income levels	Increase investment in disabled sport to make it more affordable
Poor access to facilities, poor access in and around them	Provide transport to facilities; improve access in and around them
Low levels of media coverage, few role models	Increase media coverage of disabled sport, e.g. Paralympics
Low levels of funding	Increase funding from the National Lottery
Few competitions and clubs	More competitions at all levels; more clubs for the disabled in a wider variety of sports
Myths and stereotypes	Educate people about the myths concerning disabled individuals and challenge inappropriate attitudes

Disability Sport England (**www.dse.org.uk**) is a specialist organisation involved in trying to increase participation among people with disabilities.

For disabled individuals, the benefits of participating in sport include:

- raised levels of confidence and self-esteem
- improved levels of physical skill
- increased health and fitness
- inclusion and integration into society
- more role models to encourage participation
- reducing myths and stereotypes about the disabled

Social class

Social class refers to income, background, social status and education. Playing and watching sport costs money. The more money a person has, the greater the opportunity to take part in or to watch sports.

A three-tier society is still broadly in evidence in the UK today and can be linked to sporting participation as follows:

- upper class — polo, equestrianism and field sports
- middle class — hockey, tennis, golf and rugby union
- working class — football, darts, snooker and rugby league

There is evidence that people with lower socioeconomic status participate less in sport. This is attributed to factors such as cost, lower levels of health and fitness, low self-esteem and lack of opportunities to take up sport or to become role models in positions of responsibility. People from lower socioeconomic backgrounds are more likely to suffer from social exclusion as they have less power, income and self-confidence.

Subsidised provision to encourage participation in local community schemes can help to overcome these barriers, for example Sport Action Zones set up by Sport England in some inner city areas. Such schemes also serve important functions as diversions from crime and general social disorder.

Examiner tip

In this 'Opportunities for participation' section, you might come across a 'discuss' question, e.g. 'Discuss the reasons for and against the suggestion that equality of opportunity applies to disabled people's participation in sport'. This will require you to present both sides of an argument.

Summary

By the end of this section, you should be able to:
- understand and define:
  - equal opportunity
  - discrimination
  - stereotyping
  - inclusiveness
  - prejudice
- identify the barriers to participation for various target groups, including gender, ethnicity, disability and socioeconomic class, and suggest solutions to overcome discrimination and raise participation

Questions & Answers

The specification

Unit 1 is about the opportunities for, and the effects of, leading a healthy and active lifestyle. The specification describes the aspects of PE that you need to learn. If you do not have a copy of the specification, ask your teacher for one or download it from the AQA website, **www.aqa.org.uk**. The examiners will pay careful attention to the specification when setting questions for the AS exam. If it is not in the specification, it will not be examined. If it is in the specification, it *could* be examined.

In addition to describing the content of the course (which sometimes provides detail that could earn you marks), the specification gives information about the unit tests and about other skills required — for example, using the experience gained by performing practical activities as a basis for improving physiological and psychological understanding. You also need to develop the skills of interpreting and drawing graphs and diagrams.

In addition to looking at the specification, it would be useful for you to read the examiners' reports and mark schemes from previous Unit 1 tests (these are available from AQA). These documents show the depth of knowledge that examiners are looking for, as well as pointing out common mistakes and providing advice on how to achieve good grades.

The unit test

The Unit 1 test consists of seven *compulsory* questions. There is no choice of question you have to answer all seven of them. You will have 2 hours to try to earn a maximum of 84 marks, which count for 60% of the total AS marks.

Section A is divided into three sections — applied exercise physiology, skill acquisition and opportunities for participation. There are two questions in each section. Each question is structured and worth 12 marks. Section B comprises one extended structured question, which is also worth 12 marks. The key difference for the Section B question is that it will be marked according to 'banded statements'. You will be asked a question that has two parts: an anatomy section and a skill section. Your answer will be marked by an examiner using banded marking. This will include an assessment of the quality of your written communication (QWC) as well as appropriate subject knowledge. The more responses you give from the mark scheme, the higher the band will be. Table 27 shows how the marks are allocated in relation to what number of correct points you need to 'fit into' each progressive 'band':

Table 27

Number of correct responses from the mark scheme	Level achieved	Discriminator	Initial mark awarded	QWC	Potential final mark
0			0		0
<4	1− 1+	1 or 2 points 3 or 4 points	1 2	+1 +1	1 or 2 2 or 3

5–8	2– 2+	5 or 6 points 7 or 8 points	4 5	+1 +1	4 or 5 5 or 6
9–12	3– 3+	9 or 10 points 11 or 12 points	7 8	+1 +1	7 or 8 8 or 9
13+	4– 4+	13 or 14 points 15+ points	10 11	+1 +1	10 or 11 11 or 12

It is important to write clearly in the spaces provided within the answer booklet. Avoid writing anything that you want to be marked in the margins because it might not be seen by the examiner if the paper is scanned for online marking.

There are a number of command words and terms commonly used in unit tests. It is important that you understand the meaning of each of these terms and that you answer the question appropriately.

- **Analyse/critically evaluate** — put both sides of an argument or debate, stating your opinions as appropriate.
- **Apply/demonstrate knowledge** — use practical sporting examples to illustrate clearly your understanding of theoretical content.
- **Benefits** — positive outcomes.
- **Characteristics** — features or key distinguishing qualities.
- **Define** — give a clear, concise statement, outlining what is meant by a particular term.
- **Describe** — provide an accurate account of the main points in relation to the task set.
- **Explain** — give reasons to justify statements and opinions given in your answer.
- **State/give/list/identify** — show clear understanding of key characteristics.

Whatever the question style, you must read the wording carefully, underline or highlight key words or phrases, think about your response and allocate time according to the number of marks available.

Sample questions

This section of the guide contains questions that are similar in style to those you can expect to see in the Unit 1 exam. The questions cover all the areas of the specification identified in the Content Guidance section.

Each question is followed by an average or poor response (student A) and an A-grade response (student B).

You should try to answer these questions yourself, so that you can compare your answers with the students' responses. In this way, you should be able to identify your strengths and weaknesses in both subject knowledge and exam technique.

Examiner's comments on the questions are preceded by the icon ⓔ. They offer advice on what you need to do to gain full marks. Examiner's comments on the answers are preceded by the icon ⓔ and indicate where credit is due. In the weaker answers, they also point out areas for improvement, specific problems and common errors, such as vagueness, irrelevance and misinterpretation of the question.

AQA AS Physical Education

Section A Structured questions

Applied exercise physiology

Question 1

Health, exercise and fitness

> **(a) Identify two components of fitness that are required by a sprint
> swimmer. Give an example of how one of these components is used in a race.** (3 marks)

ⓔ Make sure you identify *two* components of fitness as well as explaining how *one* of them is
used in the race.

> **(b) In a football game it is important for the performer to be fit and healthy. What do you understand
> by the terms fitness and health? Discuss whether you must be healthy in order to be fit.** (3 marks)

Total: 6 marks

ⓔ Make sure you give two definitions as well as looking at the link between health and fitness.

Student A

(a) Speed ✔ and reaction time ✔

ⓔ **2/3 marks awarded** Having correctly identified two fitness components required by a
sprint swimmer, the student forgets to say how one of these components is used during a race.
Always read the question carefully and check your answer. Look at the number of marks available
— this indicates the number of points you need to make.

Student B

(a) Speed ✔ and power ✔. Power is needed to get off the blocks with as much force
as possible ✔.

ⓔ **3/3 marks awarded** The student correctly names two relevant fitness components
required by a sprint swimmer and then says when one of these is important in a race. Always
choose the fitness components that are most relevant to the sporting activity asked for.

Student A

(b) Fitness is the ability to cope with the demands of the environment ✔ and being
healthy means having a good social, mental and physical wellbeing ✔. Fitness is to
do with the components such as speed and reaction time, whereas health is more
medical.

e **2/3 marks awarded** The student correctly defines health and fitness but fails to understand the link between them.

Student B

(b) Fitness is the ability to complete everyday tasks without fatigue ✔ and healthy is a complete physical, social and mental wellbeing, not merely the absence of disease and infirmity ✔. A performer can be fit and healthy ✔ and fit and unhealthy ✔.

e **3/3 marks awarded** Student B gives more detailed definitions and has correctly identified the link between health and fitness. Although there are four marking points in this answer, only the maximum 3 marks can be awarded.

Question 2

Nutrition

(a) **Eating a diet with sufficient calcium and iron has physiological benefits for an athlete. State the importance of these two minerals for the athlete.** (3 marks)

e Make sure you explain the physiological benefits of both calcium and iron. The question is worth 3 marks, so just stating one benefit for each will only allow you to obtain 2 marks.

(b) **In what ways should the diet of a long-distance runner be different from that of a weightlifter? Give reasons for your answer.** (3 marks)

Total: 6 marks

e You need to state what each type of performer eats and explain why.

Student A

(a) Calcium is good for bones ✔ and iron helps produce haemoglobin ✔.

e **2/3 marks awarded** The physiological benefits of calcium and iron are stated correctly but this information has not been related to the athlete. Weaker candidates often forget to apply their knowledge.

Student B

(a) Calcium is good for bones ✔ and is important for nerve transmission and muscle contraction ✔. Iron is beneficial in the production of red blood cells ✔ and this will improve the transportation of oxygen in the athlete ✔.

e **3/3 marks awarded** The student explains the benefits of calcium and iron and then relates their importance to the athlete. Four points are made but the maximum score allowed is 3 marks.

AQA AS Physical Education

Some questions do not specifically ask for definitions but including them or giving an explanation can score marks. This is a thorough answer.

Student A

(b) A long-distance runner requires more carbohydrates ✔ and a weightlifter needs more protein ✔.

ⓔ **2/3 marks awarded**   A common mistake is made here. Candidates often answer the first part of a question and forget to answer the second part. Always check your work when you have finished to see if you have missed any answers.

Student B

(b) A long-distance runner uses carbohydrate ✔ for energy ✔ and a weightlifter uses protein ✔ for muscle growth and repair ✔.

ⓔ **3/3 marks awarded** The student has answered both parts of the question correctly and has made more points than there are marks allowed.

Question 3

Pulmonary function

(a) During exercise, the oxyhaemoglobin curve shifts to the right. Explain the causes of this change and identify the effect this has on oxygen delivery to the muscles.   (4 marks)

ⓔ There are two answers to consider here, the causes of the change and the effects on oxygen delivery. Make sure you address both!

(b) The breathing characteristics of games players alter during performance. The table shows the percentages of oxygen and carbon dioxide breathed out during exercise compared with at rest.

	Inhaled air	Exhaled air (quiet breathing)	Exhaled air (exercise)
Oxygen (%)	21	17	15
Carbon dioxide (%)	0.04	4	6

Use information from the table to describe the effects of exercise on gas exchange in the lungs. Suggest why these changes occur.   (3 marks)

ⓔ Make sure you use the values from the table when you answer this question.

(c) **Explain how the increase in breathing rate experienced during exercise is controlled.** (4 marks)

Total: 11 marks

ⓔ A question on 'control' usually refers to the brain, so you need to address neural control.

Student A

(a) The curve shifts to the right because the muscles need more oxygen. This is called the Bohr shift ✔

ⓔ **1/4 marks awarded** This question appears regularly in some format and many candidates have difficulty in answering it. Try to learn two or three causes, and remember that the curve shifts to the right not because the muscles need more oxygen but because more oxygen is being released. Make sure you understand the difference.

Student B

(a) When the curve moves to the right, it is called the Bohr shift ✔. It is caused by an increase in blood temperature ✔ and carbon dioxide ✔. This means that more oxygen is released to the muscle more quickly ✔.

ⓔ **4/4 marks awarded** This is a clear, logically structured answer that scores full marks. An increase in the acidity of blood is another cause that could be given.

Student A

(b) From the table there is more oxygen consumed. This is because it is needed for energy ✔.

ⓔ **1/3 marks awarded** This question requires candidates to look at the whole table, so an answer that mentions just one gas will automatically lose 1 mark. The student should also have referred to carbon dioxide. The fact that she has only mentioned oxygen affects the second part of the answer too, and a second mark is lost.

Student B

(b) From the table it can be seen that less oxygen and more carbon dioxide is exhaled during exercise than during quiet breathing ✔. This is because oxygen is used for energy in the working muscles during exercise ✔. Carbon dioxide is a waste product of aerobic respiration ✔.

ⓔ **3/3 marks awarded** This response is detailed and covers all parts of the question. When a table is presented in a question, make sure that you refer to it comprehensively.

Student A

(c) During exercise there is an increase in carbon dioxide in the blood ✔. As a result impulses are sent to the medulla ✔ and this sends impulses to the lungs to increase breathing rate.

AQA AS Physical Education

ⓔ **2/4 marks awarded** With a little more detail, this answer could have gained full marks. The student identifies an increase in carbon dioxide but does not say that this is detected by chemoreceptors. Saying that an impulse goes to the lungs is almost correct, but you should know exactly where the impulses are sent, i.e. to the respiratory muscles. Always give as much detail as possible.

Student B

(c) There is an increase in the production of carbon dioxide ✔ and therefore blood acidity ✔. This is detected by chemoreceptors ✔. Impulses are sent to the respiratory centre located in the medulla ✔, which in turn sends impulses to the diaphragm and to the external intercostals ✔.

ⓔ **4/4 marks awarded** This student makes five correct points, one more than the number of marks allocated. Generally, with questions that do not specify a particular number, it is good exam technique to look at the mark allocation and make more points than there are marks available, in an attempt to ensure the possibility of a maximum mark. However, if a question specifies a number (e.g. 'Give two…'), only the first two answers will be marked.

Question 4

Transport of blood gases

Explain how blood flow is redistributed to the working muscles.   (3 marks)

Total: 3 marks

ⓔ The key word is 'redistributed'. In your answer, you need to explain how more blood gets to the working muscles.

Student A

Blood needs to be redistributed to the working muscles because they need more oxygen for energy.

ⓔ **0/3 marks awarded** This answer fails to score. A common error made by candidates with this question is to explain *why* blood is redistributed to the working muscles and not *how*. Always read the question carefully and highlight the words that indicate the requirements of the question.

Student B

An increase in carbon dioxide ✔ is detected by chemoreceptors ✔. An impulse is then sent to the medulla ✔ and vasodilation in the arterioles leading to the working muscles occurs ✔. Vasoconstriction also takes place in the arterioles leading to the non-essential organs ✔.

ⓔ **3/3 marks awarded** This is a detailed answer and correct terminology is used, but most importantly the student has explained *how* redistribution takes place. Including an explanation of pre-capillary sphincters could also gain a mark.

Question 5

Cardiac function

(a) Heart rate and stroke volume both increase during exercise. What causes the increase in stroke volume?

(2 marks)

ⓔ This question wants you to only state the factors that cause an increase in *stroke volume*.

(b) The heart rate increases before and during exercise and then decreases after exercise. Explain how these changes in heart rate occur.

(4 marks)

Total: 6 marks

ⓔ This answer is worth 4 marks. Make sure you address all three stages of exercise: before, during and after exercise.

Student A

(a) An increase in stroke volume is caused by an increase in venous return ✔, which means more blood can be pumped out of the heart.

ⓔ **1/2 marks awarded** Only 1 mark can be awarded because the mark scheme classes these two points made as similar — one is the result of the other. If the student had made more points than the number of marks allocated, both marks might have been gained.

Student B

(a) An increase in stroke volume is caused by an increase in the strength of contraction of the heart ✔. This means more blood can be ejected by the heart ✔.

ⓔ **2/2 marks awarded** This answer gives two correct responses and scores both marks. The student could have said that an increase in stroke volume is also caused by adrenaline and by nervous control.

Student A

(b) Adrenaline causes an increase in heart rate before exercise ✔. During exercise, receptors detect changes, such as an increase in carbon dioxide ✔. They send impulses to the brain, which increase heart rate.

ⓔ **2/4 marks awarded** Student A does not specify chemoreceptors and loses a mark. 'Brain' is too vague to score — the student should have mentioned the cardiac centre or medulla oblongata.

AQA AS Physical Education

Similarly, the SA node should have been cited, rather than simply 'heart'. Also, no explanation is given for 'after exercise'. The lack of detail in this mediocre answer means that the student scores only 2 marks.

Student B

(b) An increase in heart rate prior to exercise is due to adrenaline ✔. During exercise, there is an increase in carbon dioxide ✔ and therefore an increase in acidity ✔. This is detected by chemoreceptors ✔ and an impulse is sent to the cardiac centre ✔. This in turn sends an impulse to the SA node to increase heart rate ✔. After exercise, the parasympathetic nervous system decreases heart rate ✔.

🅮 **4/4 marks awarded** This comprehensive answer easily scores all 4 marks. The student has covered several more points than there are marks available. This is good exam technique if the nature of the question allows you to do this.

Question 6

Analysis of movement

(a) The preparation phase for the jump shown in the diagram involves a downward movement.

Complete the table to show the types of joint and joint action involved, the main agonist and the type of contraction that occurs during this downward phase.

	Type of joint	Joint action	Agonist	Type of contraction
Hip		Flexion		
Knee				Eccentric
Ankle	Hinge			

(9 marks)

🅮 Make sure you complete all parts of the table in your answer.

Questions & Answers

(b) With reference to the knee joint of the kicking leg of the footballer:

(i)   Name the articulating bones.   (1 mark)
(ii) At the moment leading up to impact, what joint action is taking place at the
      knee joint and what is the name of the agonist causing this action?   (2 marks)

ⓔ Take care when answering part (i) — there are only two articulating bones in the knee joint.

(c) Name the lever system that operates at the elbow during flexion. Sketch and label a diagram to show this type of lever.   (3 marks)

Total: 15 marks

ⓔ Remember that all lever systems in the body for the movements required by AQA involve a *third*-order lever, with the exception of extension of the elbow (first-order lever) and plantarflexion of the ankle (second-order lever).

Student A

(a)

	Type of joint	Joint action	Agonist	Type of contraction
Hip	Ball and socket ✔	Flexion	Gluteus maximus ✔	Isotonic ✔
Knee	Hinge ✔	Flexion ✔	Quads	Eccentric
Ankle	Hinge	Flexion	Gastrocnemius ✔	Isotonic

ⓔ **6/9 marks awarded** This response lacks sufficient detail. You must be specific. The movement in the ankle joint is *dorsiflexion* — flexion will not score the mark. Abbreviating muscle names will also prevent a mark being awarded — for example, 'quads' is not an acceptable answer, whereas 'quadriceps' is. Similarly, you need to be specific about the type of muscle contraction. By using 'isotonic' twice, student A is limited to 1 mark. To gain both the available marks for contraction, the student should have given the *type* of isotonic contraction, i.e. eccentric.

88   AQA AS Physical Education

Student B

(a)

	Type of joint	Joint action	Agonist	Type of contraction
Hip	Ball and socket ✔	Flexion	Gluteus maximus ✔	Eccentric ✔
Knee	Hinge ✔	Flexion ✔	Quadriceps ✔	Eccentric
Ankle	Hinge	Dorsiflexion ✔	Gastrocnemius ✔	Eccentric ✔

ⓔ **9/9 marks awarded** There is 1 mark available for each correct answer in the table. The student has correctly identified the types of joint, the joint actions, the muscles involved and the types of contraction, and so scores all 9 marks.

Student A

(b) (i) Femur and fibula.
　　(ii) The movement is extension ✔ and the agonists are the hamstrings.

ⓔ **1/3 marks awarded** One common mistake that candidates make is to name the fibula as one of the articulating bones of the knee joint. This bone actually stops before it reaches the knee. Both bones need to be correctly identified to score the mark. Candidates also often confuse the movement produced by the hamstrings and the quadriceps. This is an easy mark lost. With more revision, student A would have remembered that the hamstrings flex the knee and the quadriceps extend the knee.

Student B

(b) (i) Femur and tibia ✔
　　(ii) The joint action is extension ✔ and the agonist is the quadriceps ✔.

ⓔ **3/3 marks awarded** This is a top-level answer. All the bones, movement and muscles are correctly identified. Thorough revision of the sporting actions required by the specification will ensure success.

Student A

(c) This is a third-order lever ✔.

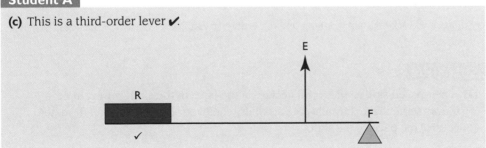

ⓔ **1/3 marks awarded** The student clearly knows the correct answer but has used abbreviations. This means that 2 marks are lost. Make sure you check all your answers, so that you do not lose easy marks.

Student B

(c) This is a third-order lever ✔.

Effort

Resistance ✔

Fulcrum ✔

ⓔ **3/3 marks awarded** The type of lever is correctly identified and the diagram is fully labelled in the correct order.

Skill acquisition

Question 7

Classification of skills

(a) Using practical examples, explain the pacing continuum. (4 marks)

ⓔ Do not use the word 'pace' in your answer! Remember to give both ends of the pacing continuum and use practical examples to illustrate your answer. The examiner should be able to easily identify which end of the continuum your example is illustrating — do not give examples that might appear in the middle of the continuum.

(b) Classify the front crawl on the continuity and muscular involvement continua and justify your answer. (2 marks)

Total: 6 marks

ⓔ Ensure you address *both* continua and remember to justify your answer — just classifying is not enough.

Student A

(a) A self-paced skill is when you decide on the pace of the skill. For example, a tennis serve. An externally paced skill is when your opponent or team-mates control the pace of the skill.

ⓔ **0/4 marks awarded** This is a weak answer. The student repeats the question by using the word 'pace'. In order to score, you must use an alternative word, such as 'rate', 'timing' or 'speed'. A tennis serve is a self-paced skill but the description is too vague to be given credit.

Student B

(a) The pacing continuum describes who controls the timing and speed of the skill ✔. A cartwheel is a self-paced skill ✔ because the performer dictates when and how fast the skill is performed ✔. Receiving a pass in rugby is an externally paced skill ✔ because the performer cannot control how fast the ball is thrown ✔ to him/her.

ⓔ **4/4 marks awarded** This is an excellent answer. It explains the continuum and then goes on to describe the extremes of the continuum. Practical examples are given for the extremes and these are very clear, ensuring the examiner will give credit.

Student A

(b) Front crawl is continuous ✔ and gross.

ⓔ **1/2 marks awarded** Student A has correctly classified the skill but has not justified the reasons for this. In this case, it is usual for a sub-maximum mark to be placed on the answer. Without justification, only 1 mark can be awarded.

Student B

(b) The front crawl is a continuous skill because it has no clear start and stop ✔. It is a cycle where the end of one stroke is the beginning of the next. It is also a gross skill because it uses a lot of large ✔ muscles in the body.

ⓔ **2/2 marks awarded** This is an excellent answer that addresses both parts of the question. The easiest way to justify anything is to use the word 'because'.

Question 8

Abilities

(a) Give two characteristics of ability. (2 marks)

ⓔ Remember to give *two* characteristics. Do not mix these up with characteristics of skilful performance.

(b) What are gross motor ability and psychomotor ability? Use practical examples to illustrate your answer. (4 marks)

Total: 6 marks

ⓔ Ensure you define both gross motor and psychomotor abilities. The examples should show how the ability is used in a sporting context.

Student A

(a) Abilities are genetically determined ✔. We get our abilities from our parents. They are stable.

ⓔ **1/2 marks awarded** The question specifies the number of answers required, so only the first two points will be marked, in this case, 'genetically determined' and 'from our parents'. Although both of these are correct, they appear on the same mark-scheme point, and therefore only worthy of 1 mark. The next point is correct but cannot be marked. Make sure your answers are clearly separate.

Student B

(a) Abilities are the building blocks of skills ✔. Abilities are stable ✔.

ⓔ **2/2 marks awarded** This student has answered succinctly and correctly, therefore scores both marks.

Student A

(b) Gross motor ability is using our innate abilities to physically perform a movement ✔ using several muscle groups. For example, strength. Psychomotor ability is reaction time.

ⓔ **1/4 marks awarded** This is a weak answer. The description of gross motor ability is well written and scores a mark, but the example is vague. The student should have stated that strength is used when performing a power lift, for example. Identifying a motor ability alone is not enough. Reaction time is a psychomotor ability but there is no clear explanation.

Student B

(b) Gross motor ability is a performer's natural ability when performing physical movements ✔ using many muscles in the body. For example, using your stamina in a marathon ✔. Psychomotor ability is about linking the mind with the body. It is when a performer processes information quickly and puts their decisions into action ✔. For example, when you judge how fast a football is being passed to you and you move closer towards it as it is slow ✔.

ⓔ **4/4 marks awarded** This is a good attempt to answer a question that candidates often have difficulty with. The examples are clear enough to gain marks. In some cases, this question would be worth only 2 marks in total, so here both the explanation and the example must be credit-worthy.

Question 9

Stages of learning

(a) Using practical examples, describe the three phases of learning. (6 marks)

ⓔ Remember to describe characteristics of all three phases of learning. Just identifying the phase will not be enough. Your practical example should link to the characteristic you have given.

(b) What are the functions of feedback? (3 marks)

Total: 9 marks

ⓔ Do not describe types of feedback. The question wants to know about *functions* — what is the role/job of feedback?

Student A

(a) Phase one is the beginners. They are slow and always have to look down and focus on the ball in basketball ✔. Phase two is intermediates. They can look up to pass and make fewer mistakes. Phase three is the experts. They are smooth when passing ✔.

ⓔ **2/6 marks awarded** This 6-mark question requires much more detail. The student has offered some correct descriptions and examples but much more time should be given to this relatively straightforward question.

Student B

(a) The first phase of learning is the cognitive phase. Movements are jerky ✔ and the learner makes a lot of mistakes ✔. When dribbling, a hockey player will start and stop and lose the ball several times.
　　In the second stage, the hockey player will start to notice that he is making mistakes and change ✔ his body or grip to rectify it. He will begin to develop kinaesthesis ✔ and know how dribbling should feel.
　　In the final stage, the performers are known as autonomous. They are experts. When dribbling they are fluent ✔ and make few mistakes. They can focus on their position on the field and where to run to next ✔.

ⓔ **6/6 marks awarded** This answer shows great exam technique. The student has given clear examples throughout. By using the same example, the three phases are clearly distinguished. The student has not identified the second phase as the associative phase, but the question does not ask for this, therefore full marks can be awarded.

Student A

(b) Intrinsic feedback comes from within. Extrinsic feedback comes from an outside source. Knowledge of performance tells you the technical information about your performance.

ℯ **0/3 marks awarded** This answer is totally irrelevant and fails to score. This is a common problem when candidates do not read the question properly. Student A has answered a question about *types* of feedback rather than *functions* of feedback. Make sure you read the question carefully and highlight the main words.

Student B

(b) Feedback tells you what you are doing correctly ✔ and detects errors ✔. If a coach tells you that you are doing something correctly, it raises your confidence ✔ and motivates ✔ you. For example, when you perform a tennis serve correctly, the coach will say, 'Well done, good speed in the serve'.

ℯ **3/3 marks awarded** This is an excellent answer. It gives more points than there are marks available and gives a practical example although it is not asked for in the question. This is good practice. There is some repetition regarding feedback informing you of correct actions — this will not gain further marks but the student will not be penalised.

Question 10

Information processing

(a) What is selective attention and why is it important for the short-term memory?   (3 marks)

ℯ Remember to answer both parts of the question. Do not describe the short-term memory store alone — the question asks why selective attention is important to it.

(b) Define reaction time, movement time and response time, using practical examples.   (3 marks)

ℯ Ensure you give concise definitions and do not use the question words in your answer. Make sure that you use a clear example for each. The 100 m sprint is probably the easiest practical example to use.

(c) One way of outwitting opponents is by 'selling a dummy'. Explain this in terms of the psychological refractory period.   (5 marks)

Total: 11 marks

ℯ Try to split the PRP into the different phases and explain what happens during the 'dummy'. The question is not asking about Hick's law!

Student A

(a) Selective attention is when a performer blocks out the crowd and focuses on just the ball ✔. It is important because the short-term memory can only hold between five and nine items ✔. The short-term memory only lasts between 15 and 30 seconds.

🄮 **2/3 marks awarded**   Both parts of the question have been addressed. Often candidates fail to do so with such questions. Student A has not given a clear definition of selective attention, but the attempt through an example would probably allow her to access the mark. She has given clear reasons for the importance of selective attention to the short-term memory. The points about the amount and length of storage are both correct but are the same points on the mark scheme and therefore gain only 1 mark.

Student B

(a) Selective attention is filtering the relevant information from the irrelevant ✔. For example, in rugby the player will focus on the ball and the incoming tackler rather than the rest of the players on the pitch and the spectators. The short-term memory has a limited capacity of five to nine items ✔ and therefore selective attention prevents information overload as it filters away the irrelevant items such as the crowd ✔.

🄮 **3/3 marks awarded** This is a good answer where both parts of the question have been addressed. Selective attention has been clearly defined and reinforced with an example. Only 1 mark is available for this part of the question, but this shows the examiner that the student has the relevant knowledge and can apply it to a practical situation. The importance of selective attention is clearly discussed, again with the help of a practical example.

Student A

(b) Reaction time is from when the stimulus is first seen or heard to when you start to move, e.g. from when the swimmer hears the starter's beep to when they dive in ✔. Movement time is the time of the whole movement, e.g. performing the dive. Response time is reaction time plus movement time.

🄮 **1/3 marks awarded** The student attempts to address all three parts of the question. Although a little vague, credit would be awarded for the answer about reaction time. The answer about movement time repeats the question and the example is vague. Response time is a combination of reaction and movement time — however, no practical example is given.

Student B

(b) Reaction time is the time from the onset of the stimulus to the onset of the response. For example, in the 100 m, this is from the gun being shot to the sprinter pushing on the blocks ✔. Movement time is the onset of the response to the completion of the task. In the 100 m, this will be from when the performer pushes on the blocks to when he/she crosses the finish line ✔. Response time is from the onset of the stimulus to the completion of the task. In the 100 m, this will be from the gun shot to the sprinter crossing the line ✔.

ⓔ **3/3 marks awarded** Student B scores 3 marks for this succinct and word-perfect answer. He has addressed all three parts of the question and given a clear practical example for each. The sprint start example is usually the easiest to describe.

Student A

(c) When you 'sell a dummy', you go one way then change your mind and go the other. This is the psychological refractory period.

ⓔ **0/5 marks awarded** This answer is far too brief for a 5-mark question. It does not say what the psychological refractory period is — it just repeats the question. Although it describes a dummy, it does not expand on this in terms of linking the theory with the practical. Student A fails to score.

Student B

(c) The psychological refractory period occurs when a second stimulus arrives before the first stimulus has been processed ✔. This is because the brain can only process one item at a time and causes the performer to freeze. In rugby, the first stimulus from the attacker would be to pretend to pass to the right ✔. The first response from the defender would be to follow ✔ the pass. The attacker would then dummy ✔ and go left, which is the second stimulus. The defender then freezes before changing direction ✔ and going to the left. This is the PRP.

ⓔ **5/5 marks awarded** This is an excellent answer. The student has answered the question fully and given a correct practical example.

Opportunities for participation

Question 11

The nature and characteristics of physical activities

(a) PE teachers aim to develop their pupils' knowledge and values. Identify values and benefits to be gained from a positive school PE experience. (4 marks)

ⓔ Try to state as many aims of PE as possible as these link to the 'positive outcomes' that the question is asking for.

(b) Play is often considered to be an educational experience. What can children learn through play? (4 marks)

ⓔ Identify a variety of different ways in which children develop as a result of play.

(c) What are the main characteristics of sport?   (5 marks)

ⓔ Try to state a variety of different features that help us categorise an activity as sport.

**(d) Apart from games, identify all other areas of activity within the
    National Curriculum for PE.**   (3 marks)

                                        Total: 16 marks

ⓔ Making sure you avoid stating 'games' as a National Curriculum area of activity, identify as many of the others as possible.

Student A

(a) Having a positive PE experience may encourage you to take up sport when you are older ✔. This can improve your health and general wellbeing ✔. Having a good experience can also help encourage young children to participate in sport.

ⓔ **2/4 marks awarded** The first two sentences earn marks as they are linked to the 'preparation for leisure' and 'improved health' values of PE. The final sentence is vague and too similar to the first point to earn another mark. The answer is too brief and lacks a range of different points.

Student B

(a) A positive PE experience can lead to:
  - the development of physical skills ✔
  - health benefits ✔
  - knowledge of the rules of a sport ✔
  - help in getting a job or career in sport ✔
  - an improvement in self-confidence ✔
  - making friends and improving social skills ✔

ⓔ **4/4 marks awarded** All six points are worth a mark. This answer is written in an examiner-friendly way with a brief introduction and the key points listed as bullets. More points have been made than there are marks available, to try to ensure full marks are earned.

Student A

(b) Children can learn how to play fairly and respect the rules of a game ✔. They can learn about sportsmanship and accepting defeat. They also learn basic skills, such as throwing and catching ✔.

ⓔ **2/4 marks awarded** This is an example of an answer that is factually correct but focuses too much on one point — fair play. The second sentence repeats the first, so a mark cannot

---

be awarded. Without the practical example, the 'basic skills' point may not have been awarded because 'skills' could relate to physical, mental or social development.

Student B

(b) ● Children can learn how to interact with others ✔.
  ● They learn fundamental motor skills by playing with such things as balls ✔.
  ● They learn cognitive skills by problem solving ✔.
  ● They learn how to cooperate and work together as a team ✔.
  ● When making up their own games, they learn creative skills ✔.
  ● They learn how to play safely ✔.

ⓔ **4/4 marks awarded** All six points are relevant and answer the question in a clear and succinct manner. Use of practical examples is further evidence of good exam practice, as is the fact that more points have been made than there are marks available.

Student A

(c) Sport is played professionally at high levels ✔. People such as Wayne Rooney earn lots of money from playing football for a living. He is a role model. I want to be like him because he plays at a high level for my favourite club. The skills he produces on the pitch are fantastic ✔, which again makes me want to be like him.

ⓔ **2/5 marks awarded** Although the use of practical examples to illustrate your understanding is to be encouraged, in this case too much focus on one person has limited the number of marks gained. Repeating the point about a professional playing for high rewards at a high level means only 1 mark can be gained because the characteristics are so similar. Reference to high skill levels gains a second mark. A variety of points should have been made in answer to this relatively simple question.

Student B

(c) Sport has a number of characteristics, such as:
  ● competitiveness and the will to win ✔
  ● rules ✔
  ● high fitness demands ✔
  ● governing bodies (e.g. the LTA) ✔
  ● use of specialist equipment ✔
  ● officials that make decisions

ⓔ **5/5 marks awarded** Just enough relevant points are made to gain maximum marks. The final point cannot be awarded a mark because it repeats the point about 'rules'. It would have been a good idea to make one or two more points, in case of vagueness or more repetition. Missing out on maximum marks on relatively easy questions can make a significant difference to the final grade achieved. Unless a specific number is asked for in the question, always make more points than there are marks available.

Student A

(d) In my PE lessons I play a lot of sport and different games such as football, cricket and tennis. I also do lots of running.

e **0/3 marks awarded** This answer is a vague attempt to earn a few marks despite a lack of knowledge of the areas of activity defined in the National Curriculum PE. The student should have highlighted or underlined 'Apart from games' in the question before starting to answer. This would have ensured that games were not included in the answer. If the final point about running had been linked to athletics, it would have earned a mark.

Student B

(d) National Curriculum PE has a number of different areas of activity:
- gymnastics and dance ✔
- swimming and athletics ✔
- outdoor and adventurous activities ✔

e **3/3 marks awarded** This is an examiner-friendly way of giving an answer in a relevant, clear and succinct manner. All areas of activity identified are correct, for full marks.

Question 12

Historical developments in sport and PE

(a) The physical activities offered by state elementary schools changed during the first half of the twentieth century. Describe and explain these changes. (7 marks)

e Start by outlining key state PE developments chronologically (i.e. in date order that they occurred) before explaining why the changes described occurred.

(b) Increasing participation in physical activity within a community is considered a positive act in today's egalitarian society. How do the reasons for increasing participation differ between local authority run clubs and voluntary clubs? (4 marks)

e State the different aims of the public sector compared to the voluntary sector in relation to increasing population.

(c) TOP Sport in England is an example of a primary school initiative. Describe TOP Sport. (4 marks)

Total: 15 marks

e Explain as many of the features of the Youth Sports Trust's TOP Sport programme as possible.

Student A

> **(a)** In the late nineteenth and early twentieth centuries there was a focus on drill (mainly military) ✔. As the twentieth century began, a more therapeutic approach to drill was introduced ✔. There was also recognition of different ages and sexes of children ✔. Following the Second World War, facilities were improved ✔ and a more child-centred approach was taken to teaching PE ✔.

@ **4/7 marks awarded** One part of the question — a description of changes to state PE — has been answered well and earns 4 marks. The final point would receive a mark, had the sub-maximum 4 marks not already been achieved. However, there is no *explanation* of these developments, as required by the question.

Student B

> **(a)** Military drill was initially taught to boys only ✔ as preparation for their military service ✔ and also to improve health and fitness ✔. In the early twentieth century, a more therapeutic approach, based on the Swedish system of drill, was introduced ✔. This was due to more emphasis being placed on children having fun ✔. As the twentieth century progressed there was more use of apparatus in schools ✔ and teachers were able to use their own initiative to teach ✔.

@ **7/7 marks awarded** This answer is made in a chronologically correct manner and includes relevant points that describe and explain developments in state PE in the early twentieth century.

Student A

> **(b)** Private-sector clubs, such as David Lloyd fitness centres, provide top-level facilities but can cost a lot of money. Public-sector clubs, such as local authority leisure centres, are cheaper but facilities are not as good. Voluntary-sector clubs, such as my hockey club, aim to provide good facilities to get more members ✔.

@ **1/4 marks awarded** This answer has a clear structure and is quite well written, but unfortunately it does not answer the question set. It is the start of an analysis of the differences between public, private and voluntary sectors, which focuses too much on facilities and does not relate to reasons for increasing participation.

Student B

> **(b)** Local authorities want to increase participation to improve the health of individuals ✔ and, therefore, to create a healthier society ✔. There are often benefits to the community. Voluntary clubs want to attract more members ✔ so they have a better chance of winning competitions ✔.

@ **4/4 marks awarded** This is a succinct, relevant answer. Both parts of the question are answered, producing a balanced response. With the relatively limited time available in the unit test, it is this type of concise answer that is needed to do well.

AQA AS Physical Education

Student A

(c) TOP Sport is a series of initiatives for children aged from 18 months to 18 years. These range from TOP Tots to TOP Sportsability. They aim to develop skills and fitness through schooling. As the schemes increase, more analysis and coaching becomes involved.

ⓔ **0/4 marks awarded** The points made are irrelevant and vague. The question requires a description of TOP Sport, which is one of the TOPS programmes. This should be the focus of the answer. However, the student focuses on describing the range of TOPS programmes available. To make sure that you answer the question set, it might help to highlight key words or phrases in the question before starting to write your answer.

Student B

(c) TOP Sport is supported and developed by the Youth Sport Trust ✔. It is designed to support teachers in their delivery of National Curriculum PE ✔ to 7–11-year-olds ✔. Training is provided for teachers to deliver TOP Sport ✔. Bags containing adapted sports-related equipment ✔ are given to teachers to help them deliver TOP Sport. Teaching cards with lesson ideas on them are also provided ✔.

ⓔ **4/4 marks awarded** Student B has answered the question set and included many relevant points on TOP Sport. More correct points are made than the maximum mark available, which is good exam practice.

Question 13

Historical and social influences on modern-day sport

(a) How might a person's ethnic background influence his/her participation in physical activity?   (4 marks)

ⓔ Identify a variety of different ways in which 'ethnicity' affects an individual's participation in physical activity.

(b) Apart from 'adaptations', in what other ways can the participation of people with disabilities be increased?   (3 marks)

ⓔ Focus on stating a variety of different solutions that would help solve the relative lack of participation of disabled individuals compared to the 'able bodied'.

(c) What social and economic barriers do women face today when attempting to participate in sport or physical activity?   (4 marks)

Total: 11 marks

(e) Give different reasons that explain the relative lack of participation in physical activity by women in comparison to their male counterparts.

Student A

(a) Ethnic background links to race. Race links to the colour of a person's skin. If you are from an ethnic minority group, you may take part less in sport because you may fear rejection by a sports club ✔ and have low self-esteem. This fear may be due to physical threats ✔ and abuse. Racial discrimination can lower participation levels.

(e) **2/4 marks awarded** This answer illustrates how a student can focus too much on a particular point or two. Though these are explained very well, repeating the same point does not earn marks. To gain more marks, the answer needs to cover a range of different points.

Student B

(a) People's ethnic background influences their involvement in physical activity, because racial discrimination may lower participation ✔. There may be fewer role models in certain sports ✔ but more in others to encourage participation. Higher values placed on education as opposed to sport may limit participation ✔. Lower levels of self-esteem may put off ethnic minorities from taking part in sport ✔.

(e) **4/4 marks awarded** Four relevant and sufficiently varied points are made to earn full marks.

Student A

(b) Disabled people often struggle to get around leisure centres ✔. They need lifts and ramps to help improve this situation. If television gave more time to disabled sport, it might help increase participation as more role models might be created ✔.

(e) **2/3 marks awarded** This answer addresses the question set and makes relevant points backed up with examples. All it lacks is a sufficient range of points to earn full marks.

Student B

(b) Participation by disabled people in sport could be increased by providing special times for them at leisure centres ✔. More clubs could be set up for them to join ✔, with specialist coaching provided ✔. If more media coverage was given, for example of the Paralympics, it might increase participation by the disabled ✔.

(e) **3/3 marks awarded** This is an excellent answer, which contains four relevant points to try to ensure maximum marks are gained.

Student A

(c) Women still have to look after children more than men ✔. Many sports are seen as too strenuous for women to take part in ✔. Myths and stereotypes still exist about what women can do.

🅔 **2/4 marks awarded** This answer is a little too brief and focuses purely on 'social' factors. In answer to a 'what' question, bullet point lists of social and economic factors linked to women's lack of participation in physical activity would suffice. No specific number of points is asked for, so relevant educated guesses could be made in an effort to gain more marks.

Student B

(c) • Sexual discrimination still exists in society today ✔.
   • Many males see sport as their preserve ✔.
   • Women tend to have jobs that pay them less ✔.
   • Women have less media coverage and fewer role models to aspire to ✔ and less funding and sponsorship ✔.

🅔 **4/4 marks awarded** A range of social and economic barriers affecting women's participation in sport is given. Once again, more correct points are written down than there are marks available.

Section B **Extended question**

Application of theory to a practical situation

🅔 For the extended question in Section B, you need to express your answer clearly and concisely but at the same time demonstrate a range and depth of knowledge. Spelling, punctuation and grammar are important, as is the use of technical language. This question is worth 12 marks and you need to give a balanced answer from both exercise physiology and skill acquisition to get into the top mark band.

> **You have been asked to help with the fitness training and skill development of a group of performers within an AS Physical Education class. Explain how the group should carry out a cool-down and give the physiological reasons behind completing one.**
>
> **What are the different forms of feedback available to a performer and how can feedback help an AS PE student?**

🅔 Question 7 of the PHED 1 exam starts with the same introductory sentence as outlined above. Make sure you address both parts of the question and write down as many answers as you can when completing each section.

Student A

A cool-down should include some low-intensity exercise such as running ✔, followed by stretches ✔. Doing a cool-down allows the body to recover faster. It gets rid of lactic acid ✔ and stops the blood pooling in the veins ✔. To perform a cool-down, the performer does light exercise first, followed by stretches.

ⓔ Student A has made four correct points in the 'fitness' section.

Student A

Feedback can help motivate the performer because it gives them information about their performance in the test ✔. If it's positive through praise, this also helps ✔. It would also be a good idea to get the other students who are not performing to cheer on those who are ✔. Getting a good score is a form of intrinsic feedback as the performer will feel good about themselves ✔.

ⓔ Student A has made four correct points in the 'skill' section.

ⓔ Student A gave eight answers in total, which initially scores 5/12 (see Table 27 on pages 79–80). 1 mark is awarded for QWC, which gives a total of 6/12 for this answer. Each section includes any number of responses from 8 up to 12, but a combined score of 20 in total is what is aimed for in the mark schemes for Question 7. This student simply did not make enough points to enter a higher band and gain more marks.

Student B

During a cool-down, exercise stops ✔ and low-intensity exercise takes place ✔, followed by stretching ✔. This keeps blood flow high and allows oxygen to be flushed through the muscles ✔ and heart rate remains elevated ✔. A cool-down can also remove lactic acid ✔ and keep the skeletal muscle pump working ✔.

ⓔ Student B has made seven correct points in the 'fitness' section.

Student B

Feedback can be intrinsic ✔ or extrinsic ✔. It can also be positive in the form of praise ✔ or negative through a critical comment ✔. It is possible to give feedback straight away so it is immediate ✔, or it can be delayed where it is given some considerable time later ✔. Feedback may help a performer to improve what they are doing as it develops confidence ✔. It can also correct or reinforce an action ✔.

ⓔ Student B has made eight correct points in the 'skill' section.

ⓔ This student gave 15 answers in total, which from the table scores 11/12. 1 mark is awarded for QWC, which gives a total of 12/12. Although this answer is not long, it hits a lot of points from the mark scheme concisely. Other answers could have included that the cool-down can maintain venous return, prevent blood from pooling in the veins and limit the effect of DOMS.

For feedback, further correct responses could have included knowledge of results (KR), where feedback is given about the outcome/result of the test, and knowledge of performance (KP), where information is given as feedback as to how well something was performed, regardless of the end result. However, enough relevant points are made to score well.

Knowledge check answers

1 The amount of work performed per unit of time.
2 Smoking reduces lung capacity/oxygen transport; lack of exercise reduces stamina; a poor diet may lead to being overweight or obese; alcohol affects concentration and can damage the heart.
3 Carbohydrates/glucose/glycogen and fats/triglycerides.
4 Food intake containing sufficient amounts of all the nutrients required (energy balance).
5 Heart disease/heart attacks; diabetes; high blood pressure; high cholesterol; stroke.
6 Scalenes, sternocleidomastoid and pectorals.
7 3% of oxygen dissolves in plasma, while 97% combines with haemoglobin to form oxyhaemoglobin.
8 Veins have a large lumen/large valves; arteries are elastic so they can withstand high pressure.
9 ● A cool-down keeps the muscles, and hence the skeletal muscle pump, working.
   ● The muscles continue to contract and compress the veins.
   ● Valves are always present and they prevent backflow of blood during the cool-down.
10 70% can be transported in the blood as hydrogen carbonate (bicarbonate) ions; 23% combines with haemoglobin to form carbaminohaemoglobin; 7% dissolves in plasma.
11 Blood flow must remain constant as the brain requires oxygen to maintain its function.
12 Increasing levels of carbon dioxide are detected by chemoreceptors; these send an impulse to the medulla/cardiac control centre; impulses are sent via the sympathetic system to the SAN.
13 This is a first-order lever.

14 Skill is learned, efficient, aesthetic and goal-directed, whereas ability is natural, stable, enduring and the foundation of skills.
15 Closed because it is unaffected by the environment (it remains the same); continuous because it has no clear beginning or ending — it is cyclic; gross because it requires several major muscle groups to perform it; self-paced because the speed of the stroke is determined by the performer, not the environment.
16 Perceptual: selectively attends and makes a judgement; translatory: selects motor programme; effector: sends impulses to the working muscles.
17 In the STSS (short-term sensory store).
18 The STM is also called the working memory. Its features are:
   ● Only relevant stimuli enter from the STSS.
   ● Limited storage space of 7 ± 2 items.
   ● Information is stored for up to 30 seconds.
   ● Information that is not rehearsed may be lost.
   ● Executes the motor programme.
   ● Passes information to the long-term memory.
19 Simple reaction time has one stimulus and one response, whereas choice reaction time has several stimuli and several possible responses.
20

21 The brain acts as a bottleneck. The second stimulus is presented and arrives in the performer's brain before he/she has had an opportunity to process the first stimulus.
22

23

Cognitive	Associative	Autonomous
• The learner creates a mental image • A demonstration is needed • Mental rehearsal of the skill is needed • Conscious thought is required • Trial and error is used • Many mistakes are made • Movements are jerky • The performer is reliant on extrinsic feedback	• Most remain in this phase • Practice is required • Demonstrations, positive feedback and mental rehearsal are still required • Fewer mistakes are made • Movements are smoother • The performer begins to focus attention away from the skill • Kinaesthesis begins to develop • Knowledge of results and knowledge of performance are required • Motor programmes develop and are stored in the long-term memory	• Movements are fluent, efficient and habitual • No conscious thought on the skill • The performer can concentrate on environmental stimuli • Kinaesthesis is used to correct mistakes • Negative feedback is used to correct errors • Practice and mental rehearsal are important to stay at this level

24 See Figure 21 on page 48.

25 Extrinsic motivation comes from an outside source and can be tangible, e.g. trophies, medals, money, whereas intrinsic motivation is from within for self-satisfaction, e.g. the pride of achieving a personal best swim time.

26 Positive reinforcement is endorsing a correct action so that it is repeated in the future, whereas negative reinforcement is criticising a performer for incorrect actions and then saying nothing when a correct action is shown.

27 • **Law of exercise** — the performer must practise the javelin throw.
 • **Law of effect** — the coach should praise the performer when the throw is correct and criticise him/her when it is thrown incorrectly.

 • **Law of readiness** — the performer should physically be able to throw the javelin and fully understand the components of the throw.

28 Attention, retention, motor reproduction and motivation.

29 Recall:
 • knowledge of initial conditions
 • knowledge of response specifications
 Recognition:
 • knowledge of sensory consequences
 • knowledge of response outcomes

30 Positive, negative, proactive, retroactive, bilateral and zero.

31 SMARTER.

32 Experience, fitness, motivation and number in group.

33

Command style	Reciprocal style	Problem solving or discovery style
Advantages • Used with dangerous situations • Used if time is short • Good for cognitive performers • Good for large groups	**Advantages** • Improves communication • Good for mixed ability groups • Instant feedback available	**Advantages** • Improves communication • Good for mixed ability groups • Motivational • Creativity encouraged
Disadvantages • Stops creativity • No differentiation in tasks • Chance of boredom/demotivation	**Disadvantages** • Time-consuming • Student coaches may lack experience • Instructions/demonstrations might be incorrect	**Disadvantages** • Time-consuming • Hard to give feedback • Working alone has safety implications • Incorrect techniques can be developed

34 Massed practice is continuous with no rest periods, whereas distributed practice has rest periods for mental rehearsal.

35 Verbal guidance is *instructing* how to perform, whereas visual guidance is *demonstrating* how to perform.

36 Manual guidance is physically supporting or forcing the performer into the action, whereas mechanical guidance is the use of a device or equipment to help the performer during the action.

37 Positive, negative, intrinsic, extrinsic, knowledge of performance, knowledge of results, concurrent, terminal and delayed.

38 Politically popular; increase health and fitness, therefore lessen strain on NHS; decrease crime (social control); increased numbers through to elite levels; economic benefits/job creation; equal opportunities/social integration.

39 Sport has a rigid structure (whereas play has a certain amount of flexibility, e.g. in terms of rules and times); sport involves high skill levels (whereas skill is not very important in play); sport is competitive (whereas a casual attitude is adopted in play).

40 Improved health and fitness; improved motor skills; opportunity to gain leadership responsibility/decision making; development of self-esteem; development of social skills/teamwork; preparation for active leisure; appreciation of the natural environment; increased risk awareness/health and safety awareness.

41 Provide facilities/opportunities for active leisure which are open to all/as accessible as possible to all.

42 Business/company; trade on normal profit/loss; managed by owners/employees; exclusive; (more) expensive.

43 Run by members; possibly on a trust/charitable status basis; financed by members' fees; run on profit/loss with any profit put back into the club; provide for 'grass roots' of sport; attempts to increase participation/performance standards in a sport; provides an opportunity to meet others with similar interests.

44 Increase health and fitness; increase obedience/discipline; prepare for army life/increase weapon familiarity.

45 A wider variety of activities (e.g. gymnastics/dance/games etc.); element of enjoyment/fun evident; facilities/equipment improved; different ages with different needs were increasingly catered for; more interactive/group work; more freedom given to teachers.

46 Increase health and fitness; learn physical/social skills; gain knowledge of the body in action; learn morality/teamwork/leadership; increase creativity/decision making; increase self-esteem; make choices for 'lifelong learning'.

47 Treating people differently, based on prejudice/stereotyping.

48 Racial discrimination/prejudice; lack of parental encouragement; low priority given to sport; cost/lack of finance; conflict with religion; fewer role models.

Note: **bold** page numbers refer to defined terms.